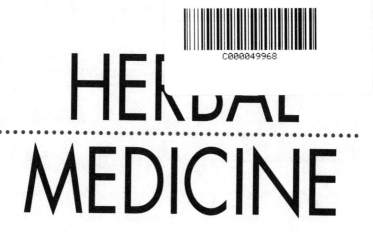

HERBAL MEDICINE

Nina Nissen

TEACH YOURSELF BOOKS

Dedication

To Li – a wise woman, my mother

For UK order queries: please contact Bookpoint Ltd, 130 Milton Park, Abingdon, Oxon OX14 4SB. Telephone: (44) 01235 827720. Fax: (44) 01235 400454. Lines are open from 9.00–18.00, Monday to Saturday, with a 24-hour message answering service. Email address: orders@bookpoint.co.uk

For U.S.A. order queries: please contact McGraw-Hill Customer Services, P.O. Box 545, Blacklick, OH 43004-0545, U.S.A. Telephone: 1-800-722-4726. Fax: 1-614-755-5645.

For Canada order queries: please contact McGraw-Hill Ryerson Ltd., 300 Water St, Whitby, Ontario L1N 9B6, Canada. Telephone: 905 430 5000. Fax: 905 430 5020.

Long renowned as the authoritative source for self-guided learning – with more than 30 million copies sold worldwide – the *Teach Yourself* series includes over 300 titles in the fields of languages, crafts, hobbies, business and education.

British Library Cataloguing in Publication Data
A catalogue record for this title is available from The British Library.

Library of Congress Catalog Card Number: On file

First published in UK 2001 by Hodder Headline Plc, 338 Euston Road, London, NW1 3BH.

First published in US 2001 by Contemporary Books, A Division of The McGraw-Hill Companies, 4255 West Touhy Avenue, Lincolnwood (Chicago), Illinois 60712–1975 U.S.A.

The 'Teach Yourself' name and logo are registered trade marks of Hodder & Stoughton Ltd.

Copyright © 2001 Nina Nissen

Typeset by Transet Limited, Coventry, England.
Printed in Great Britain for Hodder & Stoughton Educational, a division of Hodder Headline Plc, 338 Euston Road, London NW1 3BH by Cox & Wyman Ltd, Reading, Berkshire.

Impression number   10 9 8 7 6 5 4 3 2 1
Year   2007 2006 2005 2004 2003 2002 2001

CONTENTS

ACKNOWLEDGEMENTS

This book is the result of a long, exciting, and continuing journey. While the writing proved at times to be tedious, the journey was never; in a way everyone I have ever met has contributed to both.

In particular, I would like to thank the many wonderful friends who have provided meals, cups of tea, diversion, inspiration and encouragement while tolerating my absences.

To Sheila Cleary, Clare Hayden, Alice Holt and Heather Mills, who did a phenomenal job in deciphering and typing; to Joanne Ryan, whose competent corrections improved the anatomy and physiology sections; to Julie Fox for lively discussions on theory and practice; to my teachers, colleagues, clients and students who all continuously teach me so much.

Special thanks to Steive Honess who read and re-read various drafts, and whose keen eye, deep understanding of the subject matter and inspiring and tactful comments clarified many of my thoughts.

And most specially, many thanks to my son Mayo Nissen. His independence, continuous support and consideration relieved me of many of my maternal commitments and enabled me to write this book instead. Without his computer expertise, tolerance and patience, the latter stages of the writing process would have been almost impossible.

INTRODUCTION

Teach Yourself Herbal Medicine is an introduction to a vast and fascinating subject. The main objective of the book is to enable the reader actively to learn about the use of herbs in order to address common health issues.

With this aim in mind, the book is divided into three parts. In Part I, **About herbs**, herbal medicine is placed into the wider context of herbal and holistic healing and various different, yet complementary, approaches to herbs and their use are explored. This will give you a sound basis on which to make choices about the use of individual herbs, groups of herbs or herbal combinations. By drawing on your personal experiences with herbs you will be complementing and expanding on the information offered. The section on the collection and preparation of remedies will help you to decide on and prepare remedies suitable to your personal circumstances.

In general, this part offers both theoretical background knowledge and practical guidance on how to approach herbs and their many uses.

Part II, **The use of herbs**, will guide you in the practical application of herbal medicine. Herbal treatments of common health problems are outlined and this part can be used as a source for finding out about the holistic approach to individual complaints.

For reasons of clarity, information is explored according to the different bodily systems. It should enable you to identify and address minor health complaints. Suggestions made are generally applicable and appropriate in most circumstances, but are not aimed at specific and individual situations.

Part III, **The herbal**, lists 45 (mostly European) herbs in alphabetical order of their common English names. Also included are sections on actions of herbs, dosages, herbs contra-indicated in pregnancy, and ideas for working intuitively with herbs.

The herbal can be used to study a particular herb and also serves as a reference section in conjunction with the previous parts when addressing specific complaints. Should you want to collect plants from the wild, however, you will need to consult a guide book for correct identification.

As can be seen, the book can be used in several different ways. The overall aim, however, is that all parts complement and expand on each other, gradually leading to a more comprehensive understanding of the subject and a more confident and creative use of herbs.

Herbal medicine is an immensely practical subject which combines personal experiences and hands-on activities within a larger framework of holistic health and healing.

CAUTION

In the hands of an experienced practitioner herbal medicine can be used to treat serious illnesses. It should never be used in this way by anyone else. Self-diagnosis and treatment should only be used for the most minor of ailments and a doctor should be consulted immediately if symptoms persist or become aggravated.

Part I
About herbs

By way of introduction, the context of a holistic approach has been explored through assessing both an individual and empirical understanding of herbs, and the scientific knowledge gathered on the basis of chemistry and pharmacology. Drawing on information collected in such diverse ways and highlighting the many interrelationships helps to transcend historical and cultural specifics in the use of herbs, while allowing individual understanding to flourish in an encompassing paradigm. The very preparation of a simple herbal infusion is in itself a profound healing act. Combining a plant's potential with your intention, love and care facilitates change and transformation, both a cause and an effect of healing.

In order organically to draw on different experiences, while actively and practically engaging with the subject, I have juxtaposed theoretical background information with practical guidance on how to collect and prepare herbs. Hopefully, this approach will offer encouragement to experiment with herbs in a practical way and to explore the subject as widely as possible.

1 | HOLISTIC HEALTH AND HEALING

Herbal medicine is the oldest form of healing. It has been practised throughout the ages and even today the majority of the world population rely on herbs for their well-being.

Many herbal traditions, despite their differences in geography, culture, language, plants and even historical context, share a number of common concepts, the most important being a holistic approach. The word holistic has its roots in the Greek word '*holos*' – whole. It refers to integrated wholes whose parts have to be seen in relationship to the greater whole of which they are an integral part. Implicit in this concept is the need for harmony in the integration of the parts as well as harmony of each constituent yet autonomous part. It is through continuous, dynamic movement that the best conditions to create and maintain such harmony are achieved.

Within our bodies, the continuous maintenance of such balance is called homeostasis. Through homeostasis, temperature, blood pressure, electrolyte balance, hormones etc. are kept within the limits which allow for our well-being. Equally, our outer environments – our communities, the planet – have to be sustained within a framework that can actively nourish and support life, including ours. It is through observation that we can learn and understand the natural laws that govern homeostasis – from the cellular level to the planetary – and begin to live our lives again in accordance with, rather than against, them.

Integral to a holistic approach is the recognition that life, and all its manifestations, is the transformation and embodiment of energy. Depending on the tradition of healing, this energy is referred to as vital force, life force, vital spirit, vital energy or simply energy, to name but a few. The term may signify the energy of an organ, a bodily system or an individual as much as the energy of a plant, an activity, a locality, community or the cosmos.

Health is the expression of transforming energies, an inner force in continuous dynamic movement that transcends our physical well-being to include and integrate our physical body, our emotions and our mental and spiritual well-being within the wider context of our lives.

Healing and the healing process calls on the individual to embrace the flow of these energies within and surrounding us, just as the experience and expression of balance comes from within oneself. As we must consider the needs of a body system, an organ or a cell in herbal healing in the context of the whole person and her/his life, so we must integrate our health with our lives and the needs of the planet as a whole. The use of herbs can be a tool of growing awareness in this process as we explore the nature of our well-being.

Plants have been used throughout history for nourishment and healing. They offer everything our body needs for balanced and invigorated well-being. To consider herbs only as valuable sources of plant chemicals reduces their immense capacities. As an aid to the body as a whole, herbs support and strengthen our vital energies and self-healing abilities. They create an openness, the potential for change and transformation of energies which allows any necessary healing process to take place. Herbs become our allies in health and healing.

2 | UNDERSTANDING HERBS

Understanding the nature of plants is a fundamental requirement for those interested in using herbs as medicine holistically and wisely. Likewise, understanding the nature of both health and ill-health is essential in order to influence patterns of disharmony with remedies best suited to the overall situation.

Both aspects can be explored by using our individual and personal experience as a prime source of information. Here we focus on herbs; patterns of disharmony and specific diseases are the subjects of later chapters.

Throughout history the nature of herbs has been explored and described by drawing on those qualities which we can perceive through our senses. Through combining an intuitive understanding of plants with clinical experience, extensive empirical information has been collected throughout the ages. Before choosing a herb for healing explore the plant through sight, touch, smell and taste to create a picture of it. This will guide you to a discovery of its vital energies and healing potential and will also enhance your understanding. You can feel the soft quality of Mullein leaves and experience its soothing and moisturising effects in dry respiratory conditions; you can smell the stimulating aroma of Peppermint and enjoy its cooling effects as a skin lotion; you can taste the hot pungency in Ginger and immediately feel its warmth on drinking an infusion.

The taste of plants especially, as well as their qualities of warming/cooling and moisturising/drying, have consistently shown predictable therapeutic effects.

The taste of plants can be subdivided into sour, sweet, bitter, salty, pungent and bland. Each category has its specific physical, emotional or mental effects; these may be localised or general, immediate or long term. The warming or cooling (or neutral) effects of a herb are based on a plant's objective ability to be warming or cooling as well as an individual's experience of it. Many factors contribute to determining a plant's temperature: including climate, the seasons, a person's tendency to be warm or cold and the nature of the complaint. In addition, herbs have the ability to be moisturising or drying (or neutral) in their effect on the body and its tissues.

Such qualities uncover a plant's manifold layers and add depth to our understanding of its healing potential, its resulting actions and uses. In general, a condition is treated with herbs of opposite aspects to the complaint; a hot inflamed joint is cooled down, a dry cough moisturized, a runny nose dried up and cold extremities warmed. Through gathering information in this way you will learn about the unique healing potential of each plant in influencing not only physical well-being but also promoting emotional and mental balance. (See also Chapter 20 on intuitive work with herbs).

Over time, these sense-perceptible qualities have been empirically refined and further interpreted. Today, they are mostly described as the 'actions' of a herb (see Chapter 17). The interrelationships between tastes and their qualities, energies and selected actions are generalized and summarized in the following table.

Sour	Energy	prevents dispersal of energy and fluids
	Quality	cooling, drying, gathering, binding, absorbing, can be stimulating
	Effect	causes contractions, toning to tissues, reduces secretions
	Action	astringent, anti-inflammatory
Bitter	Energy	moving body energy downwards
	Quality	cooling, relaxing, stimulating, drying, balancing
	Effect	clears congestion and stagnancy and reduces overactivity and excesses, especially in the digestive system and the liver, detoxifying
	Action	bitter, tonic, laxative

Sweet	Energy	moves and expands upward and outwards
	Quality	warming, although may also be cooling, relaxing, moisturizing, especially in dry conditions, harmonizing, energizing
	Effect	soothes, restores, tones and strengthens tissues and organs; cleanses, harmonizes
	Action	demulcent, emollient, expectorant, tonic, relaxant
Pungent	Energy	moves upwards and outwards to the periphery of the body
	Quality	warming, occasionally cooling, stimulating, relaxing, calming, expansive, dispersive
	Effect	stimulates circulation of energy and blood
	Action	stimulant, relaxant, carminative, diaphoretic, expectorant
Salty	Energy	moves downwards and inwards to the centre of the body
	Quality	cooling, moisturizing, grounding, balancing, especially to fluids
	Effect	moistens dryness, softens hardened tissue, detoxifying, nourishing
	Action	diuretic, alterative, nutritive
Bland	Energy	moves downwards and outwards
	Quality	drying, balancing to temperature, neutral
	Effects	detoxifying
	Action	diuretic, nutritive

Note: Plants can and do fall into more than one category, such as bitter/sweet or sweet/sour.

Plants can exhibit different effects depending on the person and their complaints, for example Lavender can be both relaxing and stimulating, Peppermint both warming and cooling.

As you become increasingly familiar with herbs, you will gradually be able to create a holistic picture of each plant to be used with wisdom and clarity. The inclusion of scientific insight can facilitate this process and help you to understand and explain your own experience as well as the traditional empirical uses of herbs.

Our next task is to explore the chemistry and pharmacology of herbs.

3 | **KNOWING HERBS**

Plant chemistry and pharmacology

Knowledge of plant chemistry is not essential to the practice of herbal medicine, although much valuable insight can be gained to broaden our understanding of plants and explain some of their actions and empirical uses. The focus here will be on the effects of plant constituents on our body.

At no point, however, must the view of the whole be lost: it is essential to bear in mind that herbs are not used on the basis of any one constituent. Rather, all substances contribute to a plant's action and uses by complementing, enhancing, reducing and/or suppressing the various components in a blend unique to each plant.

In using the whole plant we draw on the plant's synergistic harmony encompassing more than the sum total of its individual parts.

Mucilage

Mucilages are complex carbohydrates, which produce a slimy, gel-like protective layer on the contact surface. They soothe, relax and protect the skin and mucus membranes of the digestive, respiratory and urinary systems in conditions of irritation and inflammation, they increase the fluidity of bronchial secretion and are overall cooling in effect.

They are used to soothe the gut by reducing sensitivity to gastric secretions and calming peristalsis and spasms. They relieve irritable, dry coughs and bronchial tension and ease the pain of urinary infections and inflammations.

Externally, mucilaginous plants are used in wound healing to ease pain, irritation and itching.

Action:	demulcent emollient	Taste:	sweet to bland
Example:	Comfrey Marshmallow Mullein Ribwort	Quality:	moist, cooling

Tannins

Tannins have the ability to bind with proteins on the skin and mucus membranes to form a protective layer which becomes resistant to microbial invasion and inhibits secretions. This action is referred to as astringency.

Astringent plants are used medicinally in the treatment of inflammatory digestive complaints such as gastritis, enteritis and diarrhoea, respiratory catarrh, internal bleeding and the healing of wounds, burns and infections of the eyes, mouth, gum, genitals and cervix.

Action:	anti-inflammatory antiseptic astringent	Taste:	sour
Example:	Agrimony Elderflower Horsetail Raspberry Ribwort	Quality:	drying

Flavonoids

Flavonoids are universal in plants, but they are especially present in flowers, fruits and leaves and those with yellow and white pigmentation.

The main action of the flavonoids is on the heart and circulatory system. They lower blood pressure, decrease capillary fragility, protect blood vessel walls and improve the peripheral circulation. Some flavonoids also exhibit anti-oxidant protective effects against cell damage and additional anti-inflammatory and diuretic properties.

Flavonoids act synergistically with vitamin C found together in most fruits and berries.

Action:	anti-inflammatory anti-oxidant anti-spasmodic diaphoretic diuretic	Taste:	sweet to bitter
Example:	Elderflower Hawthorn Lime flower St John's Wort Yarrow	Quality:	balancing warming to cooling

Alkaloids

Alkaloids, the most potent of all plant constituents, tend to be toxic in large amounts and are, therefore, not suitable for home use.

The actions of the many alkaloids vary considerably from one plant to another, with effects on the nervous system being the most prominent. Many modern drugs are derived from plant alkaloids and include atropine, morphine and nicotine as well as caffeine, one of the most widely occurring alkaloids.

In small, non-toxic amounts, alkaloids tend to reinforce and potentize other healing components and properties of herbs.

Action:	various	Taste:	bitter
Example:	Borage Comfrey Vervain	Quality:	cooling

Saponins

Saponins, named after their soap-like action of forming lather when mixed with water, exhibit a wide variety of therapeutic effects.

The softening and cleansing properties, in for example Oats and Marigold, can be helpful in the external treatment of skin complaints, whereas the saponins found in Mullein have a stimulating and cleansing effect on the respiratory system leading to improved expectoration; those found in Horsetail cause effective diuresis. The stimulation of the digestive system due to saponins in Oats, Horsetail and Marigold aids the absorption of minerals. Saponin-rich herbs are also prominent in the treatment of vascular disorders as they strengthen fragile blood vessels and lower blood cholesterol levels; these include Horsechestnut, Yarrow and Lime-flowers. Steroidal saponins have a hormone-like effect on the body while others are found to have a balancing effect, improving overall well-being.

Action:	adaptogenic anti-inflammatory diuretic expectorant	Taste:	sweet
Example:	Borage Horsechestnut Horsetail Limeflower Liquorice Marigold Oats Yarrow	Quality:	neutral to slightly cooling

Volatile oils

Volatile or essential oils, probably the best known plant constituent (we commonly encounter them in aromatic herbs), consist of complex chemical compounds and combinations. These give the plant not only its individual smell and taste but also its specific therapeutic activities. Nevertheless, certain aspects shared by volatile oils can be identified.

All volatile oils have a direct antiseptic and anti-microbial effect while also supporting the body's own healing capacities by increasing white blood cell production. Both internally and externally, volatile oils stimulate the tissues they come into contact with. This increases the circulation, stimulates expectoration and enhances digestive functions such as appetite, digestion and absorption as well as peristalsis. Effects on the nervous system can be both relaxing and stimulating, overall enhancing and co-ordinating functions throughout the whole body.

Given the nature of volatile oils, they lend themselves to a number of different uses. Not only do they enter the bloodstream on being taken internally, but they can also penetrate and rapidly disperse through the skin when applied externally or act on the nervous system on inhalation.

Action:	analgesic antiseptic anti-spasmodic carminative expectorant relaxant stimulant	Taste:	pungent
Example:	Garlic Ginger Lavender Peppermint Rosemary Thyme	Quality:	warming with cooling after-effect; drying

Bitter principles

The bitter principles represent a diverse group of constituents which have in common a bitter taste, often characteristic of herbal remedies.

Bitter principles initiate their therapeutic effect through the taste buds and a subsequent reflex action in the gut. They stimulate the appetite and the secretions of all digestive juices, improve digestive absorption, assimilation and elimination, enhance liver function and promote the flow of bile. Through improved digestive and liver function overall well-being is enhanced and immunity strengthened.

Traditional digestive drinks and tonics recognize that bitters naturally complement food and benefit the digestion. In holistic treatment bitters are, above all, stimulating tonics called for in a wide variety of circumstances. In order to benefit fully from the bitter principles in herbs, preparations should not be sweetened as this counteracts the bitter stimulus.

| Action: | bitter
laxative
tonic | Taste: | bitter |
| Example: | Burdock
Chamomile
Dandelion
Marigold
Peppermint
Vervain | Quality: | cooling |

Vitamins, minerals and trace elements

Essential to health and all metabolic reactions, vitamins, minerals and trace elements are found in abundance in herbs.

The nutritive action of herbs can often be noticed through a sweet to bland and/or salty taste with an overall grounding quality.

4 | MEETING THE PLANTS

Collection and drying of herbs

Before embarking on making a herb collection, take note of the plants that grow around you, between your front door and garden gate, along your way to the shops, in your local park or your favourite spot in the woods.

Try to become knowledgeable with the help of good field guides and find out if any herbalist or botanist organizes herb walks so that you can learn to recognize plants growing in the wild.

Learn about one or two plants at a time, make them your friends and allies. And even if you never gather your own plants from the wild, it is deeply satisfying to know about their personalities, what they look like and where and how they grow.

Collection

Plants will be more potent if gathered at a time when the plant's healing energy is most concentrated; this varies with different plant parts.

■ *Flowers*: gather just before or just after flowers open; collect in clear dry weather, once the dew has evaporated, but before the heat of the day sets in.

■ *Leaves and aerial parts*: gather while flowering or just before the flower fades. Collect in clear, dry weather once the dew has evaporated but before the heat of the day sets in. (Note: the term 'aerial parts' refers to all parts above ground including stems, leaves and flowers.)

■ *Seeds and berries*: collect when mature, usually late summer to autumn.

■ *Roots*: gather annuals before the plant flowers, biennials after vegetation of the last year has ended and perennials either in spring or autumn.

General points to consider

■ Choose a clean area to pick your plants, away from pollution (traffic, agriculture, domestic). Be clear when you set out what you are looking for and what you intend to prepare with your harvest so that you will gather only as much as you will need and can use at the time.

■ Gather your herbs into paper bags as this allows the plants to breathe.

■ Do not over-harvest a spot or neither you nor anyone else will be able to enjoy nature's offerings later.

■ Your respectful attitude when collecting plants is as important as the quality of the plants you gather.

■ As you have already decided what preparations you want to make, you can deal with your harvest immediately. This will preserve the plants' energies, colour, fragrance, taste and medicinal properties. Allowing the plants to lie about dissipates their energies, encourages mould and fermentation and evaporates volatile oils. Less potent preparations are the result.

Drying

If you want to dry any herbs, get them ready as soon after collection as you can.

■ *Flowers and leaves*: spread material loosely on plain paper; do not dry them in the sun, but do ensure good air circulation. Sometimes flowers and leaves can be tied into bunches and hung up in an airy place for drying (e.g. Elderflower). Large, fleshy leaves like Comfrey and Borage need stringing up individually.

■ *Aerial parts*: tie up into small bunches and hang (upside down) in an airy dry space.

■ *Seeds, berries and bark*: spread on plain paper and turn regularly until dry.

You should not need to wash any parts growing above ground.

■ *Roots*: wash thoroughly and, if large, cut into smaller pieces, lay out on plain paper and turn regularly till dry.

Storage of herbs

Dried plants are ready for storage when they are crisp and brittle to the touch. To preserve their healing qualities, they need to be stored at this point rather than looking pretty in your home while fading in energy.

If your surroundings are damp, store the herbs in paper bags which allow the plants to breathe. Otherwise, you can use glass jars.

Label your bags or jars with name and date and keep them in a dry cupboard.

Buying herbs

Knowing how to buy dried herbs is an important skill which can be learned with a little time and experience. Essentially, the herbs you buy should be intensely coloured, fragrant and as whole and unprocessed as possible.

When you look at a herb, envisage the whole plant as it is when it is growing. Marigold flowers are a vibrant yellowish-orange when in bloom and the colour should be preserved even when dried. Nettle leaves are a deep green and only turn brown and listless when wilting and old.

Smell the herb carefully: the scent and aroma should be fresh and immediately noticeable. Poorly dried, stored or old materials smell musty; roots and berries may even be mouldy. Processed herbs more often than not lose their colour and scent. If you do not recognize the fresh plant in the dried herb you should probably reject it as it will have lost its vibrant healing energy.

TIP: Compare Peppermint or Chamomile teabags with a handful of loose dried herbs.

5 | HERBAL PHARMACY

The art of making herbal preparations is fundamentally simple, yet satisfying and inspiring. As an expression of self-care or concern for others, it is imbued with your loving energy, which is a vital contribution to the healing process.

Most kitchens are equipped with the essentials needed:

- teapot and strainer
- pots and pans, preferably stainless steel, not aluminium
- jars with lids
- glass bottles with screw tops
- sharp knife and chopping board
- scales.

You may need only to buy labels so that you can identify your preparations with name and date.

Your choice of preparation may be determined by a number of variables including:

- availability of ingredients
- method and ease of preparation
- the complaint to be treated
- your confidence and experience.

However, preparing a herbal remedy is rarely more complex than basic food preparation.

Herbal medicines are commonly prepared in three bases:

- water
- alcohol
- oil.

In all bases only gentle heat is used in order to preserve or enhance the healing potential of the plant.

Water-based preparations

Water-based preparations are potent remedies with an accessible range of nutrients and healing properties which are easily digested and assimilated, especially when the user is unwell. In most situations, I prefer herbal medicines in a water base as our bodies have a close affinity with water.

Infusion

A standard preparation is suitable for flowers, leaves, aerial parts and fine roots, barks, berries and seeds.

Ingredients

- ¹/₂–1 teaspoon of dried herb/s, or
- 1–2 teaspoons of fresh herb/s
- 250 ml of boiling water

Method

- Pour the boiling water over the finely chopped herb/s.
- Cover well with a lid and leave to infuse.

Infusion times: flower: 3–4 minutes
leaves and soft aerial parts: 5 minutes
woody aerial and other fine hard parts: 5–15 minutes

- Strain and enjoy colour, aroma, flavour and effects.

Tip: Standard infusion can be drunk hot, warm, cold and iced, whereby the different temperatures contribute to different effects. For example, hot elderflower tea increases sweating, cooled or iced it is uplifting and refreshing.

Dosage: standard treatment   1 cup 3 x day

       (See also Chapter 18 on dosages)

Decoction

A standard decoction is suitable for hard plant materials (seeds, berries, roots, bark) which require longer extraction to access their healing properties.

Ingredients

■ 40g of dried herb/s or
■ 60g of fresh herb/s
■ 1 litre of boiling water

Method

■ Cover the chopped herb with boiling water.
■ Simmer very gently for 20–30 minutes.
■ Strain and enjoy colour, aroma, flavour and effects.

Tip: A decoction will keep 2–3 days in refrigerator.

Dosage: standard treatment $^{1}/_{4}$ cup 3 x day
              Dilute with water to taste

              (See also Chapter 18 on dosages)

Infusions and decoctions can also be used externally as:

■ body wash
■ hand, foot, sitz or full body bath
■ hair rinse
■ eye wash
■ gargle
■ douche
■ steam inhalation
■ poultice
■ compress

Poultice or cataplasm

Poultices are commonly applied warm or hot in order to improve local circulation, relieve spasm and tension, ease pain, reduce infections and inflammation, draw out toxins or foreign bodies and to heal bruising, swelling and wounds.

Ingredients
- damp plant material, strained out of an infusion or decoction or
- fresh plant material, grated, crushed, chewed

Method
- Place plant material directly or wrapped in thin gauze on the affected area.
- Keep in place with a cloth or cling film.

Tip: If a poultice is used hot, rub some olive oil into the affected area before application to avoid burning.

Compress or fomentation

In general hot compresses are relaxing and easing to local congestion such as cramps, aches and pains or tension. Cold compresses are toning and stimulating in, for instance, tiredness and are very effective in reducing fevers and inflammation.

Ingredients
- hot or cold water or
- hot or cold infusion or decoction

Method
- Soak a soft cloth in your chosen liquid.
- Squeeze out any excess.
- Apply to affected area.

Tip: If using a hot compress apply some olive oil to the affected area before application to avoid burning.

To keep a compress warm, place a hot water bottle over the application.

Syrups

Herbal syrups are pleasant to make, nutritive and versatile as you
can mix small quantities of tincture into a base syrup to adapt it to
your needs. Syrups can be prepared from all herbs and spices,
although syrups with antiseptic and demulcent actions such as
Ribwort, Thyme or Liquorice are especially suitable to cure
coughs, chest tightness and respiratory infections.

Ingredients
■ 40g of dried herb, or
■ 60g of fresh herb
■ 900 ml of water
■ 450g of honey or sugar
■ 1 tablespoon brandy or vodka (optional)

Method
■ Prepare a standard decoction.
■ Strain and continue to simmer very gently to reduce to at
  least half of the original fluid.
■ Add the honey or sugar and bring briefly to the boil.
■ Stir continuously and simmer until sweetener is dissolved.
■ Add brandy or vodka to stabilize the syrup (optional).
■ Store in clean, sterilized bottles. Label with name and date.

Dosage: standard treatment 2–3 teaspoons in warm water
                              3–5 x daily

(See also Chapter 18 on dosages)

Alcohol-based preparations

Tinctures

Herbs prepared in vodka, brandy, wine, vegetable glycerine or
vinegar are called tinctures, whereby the healing properties of the
plant are extracted and preserved in your chosen medium. Tinctures
are a popular preparation for both internal and external use.

Some advantages of tinctures over water-based preparations are due to the fact that a small amount of plant material produces a medicine which:

■ remains potent for many years
■ is effective in small quantities and sparing in use
■ is easily available when needed
■ is convenient, for example when travelling or taking very bitter herbs.

However, herbs are often used for the supporting and healing nourishment they offer. As only a small amount of tinctures are used, water-based preparations tend to support the body's healing with greater affinity. In addition, the ritual of preparing and drinking a herbal infusion or decoction is not only a pleasure but a healing act in itself.

Standard home tincture

Ingredients

■ 25g of dried herb or
■ 50g of fresh herb
■ 250 ml brandy, vodka, vinegar or vegetable glycerine
■ 150 ml water (boiling if using glycerine)

Method

■ Place your chopped or bruised herb in a jar.
■ Mix the fluids together and add to your herbs, making sure that all herbs are well covered with fluid.
■ Close your jar well; label with content and date.
■ Keep in a cool dark place and shake daily.
■ After 2–4 weeks, strain and squeeze the herb thoroughly through a thin cloth to obtain your tincture.

Tip: Store your tincture in dark glass bottles, label and keep in a cupboard.

Dosage: standard treatment   20 drops–1 teaspoon 3 x daily
                  (See also Chapter 18 on dosages)

Tinctures are best taken in $1/2$–1 glass of water, 15 minutes before food. If you avoid taking alcohol, dilute your tincture in warm water and allow to stand for several hours for the alcohol to evaporate before drinking. Tinctures can be diluted and used externally just like infusions or decoctions.

Oil-based preparations

Infused oils

Infused oils can be prepared by infusing a herb in a base oil of sunflower, olive, coconut, almond etc. so that the healing properties of the plant are imparted to the oil.

There are two ways of preparing infused oils.

Sun method

This method works well with delicate, aromatic plant parts, for example the flowers of Rose, Mullein, St John's Wort, Dandelion and the leaves of Lemon Balm.

Ingredients

■ Fresh aromatic leaves or flowers, chopped or bruised if needed
■ Oil of your choice to cover herb material

Method

■ Fill a glass jar with your herb.
■ Cover well with the oil, leaving no air space.
■ Cover tightly, label and leave in a sunny place for two weeks, shaking the contents regularly.
■ After two weeks, strain the herb and replace with fresh plants to increase the potency of the infused oil.
■ Repeat as often as required.
■ Should a watery residue collect at the bottom of your jar, be sure to discard this carefully as it will spoil the oil.

Tip: Store the oil in dark glass bottles, label and keep in a cool place.

Stove method

This method works well with harder plant parts, for example fresh or dried Comfrey leaves/root, Ribwort, Yarrow or Rosemary, but can also be used for any other herb.

Ingredients

■ Chopped or bruised herb
■ Oil of choice to cover the herb

Method

■ Place the herb in a small pan.
■ Cover with the oil and place a lid on.
■ Gently heat in a waterbath (*bain-marie*) for 2 hours
■ Strain well and discard the herb.
■ Repeat above steps with fresh herbs, using the same oil.
■ Should a watery residue collect at the bottom, discard it carefully.

Tip: Store the infused oil in dark glass bottles, label and keep in a cool place.

Optional: to prevent rancidity of infused oils add 5% wheatgerm oil or vitamin E (from capsules).

Ointments

Ointments are easily prepared from infused oils thickened with beeswax. They are by nature greasy, preserve water and heat and provide a protective layer, which allows healing to take place. Ointments are, therefore, used especially for delicate or rough and dry skin and deep muscular or joint pain aggravated by cold.

They should not be used in hot conditions or with weepy, inflamed skin complaints.

Marigold makes an excellent and versatile ointment, suitable for most household first aid needs.

Simple ointment

Ingredients

■ 300 ml infused oil
■ 25 mg yellow beeswax, chopped or grated

Method

■ Gently heat the infused oil in a waterbath.
■ Melt the beeswax into the oil, stirring continuously until dissolved.
■ Allow mixture to cool for a few minutes.
■ Pour into clean jars.
■ Once set and cooled, close jars with lids, label and store in a cupboard.

Part II
The use of herbs

The holistic use of herbs emphasizes the notion that health is a positive state of being, focuses on the needs of the individual and treats the whole person rather than isolated symptoms and manifestations of disease.

Information is explored in the different bodily systems whereby each system is presented within the following format:

- the holistic relevance of the bodily system under discussion
- a brief outline of its anatomy and physiology
- herbs and their categories particularly relevant to the system
- a description of minor complaints together with suggestions of herbal recipes
- additional self-help strategies such as dietary advice and lifestyle changes.

Information in this part can be used to identify and assess minor health complaints and to develop a holistic approach to individual problems. It is advisable to study further any herbal suggestions made.

- Refer to 'The herbal' to assess the individual suitability of a herb or a combination of herbs.
- Strictly follow all standard dosages given in 'The herbal'; if using herbs for children or the elderly, refer to Chapter 18 for relevant dosages.
- Adhere to contra-indications at all times.
- If symptoms persist, consult a qualified practitioner. Do not diagnose or treat serious conditions without professional advice.

Throughout, the promotion of health and the prevention of disease are seen as priorities while any therapeutic suggestions aim to support a person's self-healing capabilities and ability to take responsibility for their self-care.

6 | **THE IMMUNE SYSTEM**

The immune system plays a fundamental role in the holistic maintenance of health by combining the prevention of diseases with supporting specific healing processes in ill-health. Hence, it provides a pertinent introduction to this overview of the bodily systems by focusing attention primarily on the active maintenance of health and vitality, and only secondarily on the disruptive effects of illness and the alleviation of disease, both acute and chronic.

Through the immune system the body protects itself against potentially disease-producing micro-organisms such as viruses, bacteria, fungi and parasites and also maintains a stable internal and external physiological environment. It can be likened in structure to an onion with its many layers – the outermost skin being tough and resilient and protecting the soft, more vulnerable inner layers.

Plants can be a powerful tool in maintaining well-being as they can be used both for nutritional and medicinal purposes in harmony with the natural physiological rhythms of our body. As herbal medicine is health rather than disease oriented, its overall aim is to strengthen the person and their individual characteristics.

As we will see, a holistic approach is particularly relevant when exploring the immune system.

Anatomy and physiology

Due to the actions of a number of interrelated defence mechanisms, we only occasionally fall ill, despite being surrounded and inhabited by a multitude of microbes.

Primary organs of the immune system are:

■ Bone marrow
■ Thymus

Bone Marrow

The bone marrow contains the precursors of all lymphocytes and discharges them in various stages of maturation into the circulation. Some lymphocytes mature undergoing changes in the bone marrow to become B-lymphocytes; some undifferentiated lymphocytes migrate via the blood to the thymus to become T-lymphocytes before re-entering the circulation. Others become large lymphocytes, enter the circulation and migrate to secondary organs such as the spleen, tonsils, adenoids, appendix and assorted deep and superficial lymph nodes (see also lymphatic system).

The spleen serves as a reservoir of red blood cells processes incoming blood and may react rapidly to the presence of micro-organisms, including antibody production. It also removes old blood cells from the circulation.

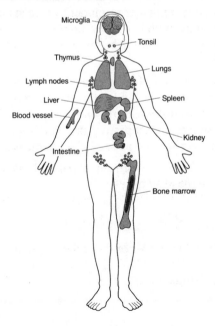

Thymus

The thymus is actively concerned with the differentiation and proliferation of T-lymphocytes received in an undifferentiated form from the bone marrow via the blood.

Natural defences

Natural defences help to maintain the body's integrity on a daily basis. Skin and mucous membranes provide a physical barrier. In addition, the skin and sweat contain anti-bacterial and anti-fungal substances and secreted mucus traps microbes on its sticky surface. Should microbes reach the stomach after contact with antiseptic saliva, the hydrochloric acid in gastric juice will destroy the majority of them. Beneficial bacteria in the intestine hold any unwanted substances in check which will then be excreted with the faeces. The urinary system flushes out any organisms with the urine and acids in the vagina destroy any organisms there. Eyes are continuously cleansed by antiseptic tears.

Sneezing, coughing, vomiting and diarrhoea are reflexes which promptly and forcibly expel any unsuitable substances be they microbes, pollutants, foreign bodies or allergens.

Inflammation

Should any of the above defences fail and microbes enter the body, the immune system responds with an inflammation. This will check microbial invasion and heal any damaged tissue.

Through extra blood flow to the affected area, the body delivers extra white blood cells, which help to remove any microbes. The affected area will become red, swollen, hot and painful and may discharge fluids such as pus or phlegm. Should the increased blood flow prove insufficient to clear the problem, more powerful white blood cells will be brought into the area. Lymphocytes, suspended in lymph fluid, will destroy microbes and collect any toxins, which then will be dealt with in the lymph nodes and other secondary immune organs. Swollen lymph glands hence indicate that your body's immune system is actively dealing with an infection.

Acquired immunity

In certain situations a more specific immune response takes place.

As a result of an invading microbe (antigen) the body produces antibodies which in future will recognize the original antigens. This enables the body to deal immediately with the specific infection without instigating a further inflammatory attack. This process is called 'having acquired immunity' or 'being immune'. It underlies many infectious childhood diseases such as measles, mumps and chickenpox which we tend to suffer from only once in our life.

Allergy

In allergy, a person becomes hypersensitive to a variety of foreign proteins ranging from natural to chemical substances, including pollen, dust mites, animal furs or foods.

An allergic response involves an exaggerated reaction of the immune system related to the release of chemicals and their action on the body.

Lining the mucous membranes are white blood cells called mast cells. These produce special antibodies with a memory, known as immunoglobulins. On repeated exposure to the same substance, immunoglobulins bind to mast cells and form a complex allergen, which attaches to cells in the blood vessels and tissues. An immediate inflammatory response occurs at the site of contact, resulting in the release of histamine and prostaglandins, among other chemicals. These cause an extremely diverse range of symptoms such as itching of the skin, watery eyes, swelling of mucous membranes, overproduction of mucus in the respiratory system, diarrhoea or constipation, headaches, lethargy, hyperactivity and many more.

In very severe cases, the inflammatory response spreads throughout the body causing extensive dilation of the blood vessels and a consequent drop in blood pressure which can be fatal. This rare condition is known as anaphylactic shock and is occasionally seen in nut allergies and as a reaction to wasp and bee stings.

Auto-immune disease

The key to our immune defences is the body's ability to differentiate between our own and foreign proteins.

Occasionally, the system becomes confused and attacks the body's own tissues causing serious and mostly chronic inflammatory diseases such as arthritis, psoriasis and multiple sclerosis. Chronic degenerative diseases may also be caused by this process.

Herbs for the immune system

Bitter tonics

Promote liver and digestive functions and are often used to improve integrated well-being:

Burdock root	Marigold
Dandelion root	Vervain

Diuretics

Increase the secretion and elimination of urine-improving detoxification:

Dandelion leaf
Nettle

Alteratives

Detoxify the blood and lymphatic system and promote the renewal of body tissue; they are often called for in recurring infections:

Cleavers	Nettle
Echinacea	Red Clover
Marigold	

Diaphoretics

Promote sweating and eliminate toxins through the skin, assisting kidney function:

Ginger	Vervain
Lime flower	Yarrow
Peppermint	

Nervine tonics

Nourish and strengthen the nervous system, thereby improving healthy function and promoting well-being and vitality. They combine well with adrenal tonics in long-standing complaints:

Lavender	Skullcap
Oats	Vervain
Rosemary	Wood Betony

Anti-microbials

Destroy, inhibit or resist disease-causing micro-organisms and help the body to defend and protect itself against disease:

Echinacea	Marigold	Thyme
Garlic	Ribwort	
Lavender	Sage	

Adrenal tonics

Help to promote the functioning and balance of the adrenal gland; they are especially relevant in times of prolonged stress and ill-health:

Borage
Ginger
Liquorice

Complaints of the immune system

A vibrant immune system is characterized by even physical and mental energy levels with a healthy emotional balance, infrequent infections and prompt recovery in case of illness. Such immunological vitality demonstrates homeostasis in continuous and dynamic action, whereby balance and harmony are the keys to well-being.

A healthy and varied diet, plenty of fluids, suitable, regular exercise and a balanced emotional and mental outlook with pleasures and relaxation, an integral part of self-care, keep our immune system healthy and active. Foods such as refined carbohydrates, especially sugar, caffeine, alcohol, processed foods, high salt intake and excessive and prolonged stresses weaken the system.

Acute conditions

Weaknesses in the skin and mucous membranes allow the entrance of microbes and their resulting damage. Superficial infections, as in acute disease such as a cut, a cold, measles, diarrhoea etc., are vigorously addressed by our bodies with often uncomfortable mechanisms in order to defend our well-being. Responses may range from a sore throat, runny nose and fever to skin eruptions, vomiting and pus-filled wounds.

Herbs can be used for their direct anti-microbial action as well as to support the body's own healing capacities. Care should be taken not to suppress the symptoms but to treat the underlying cause and strengthen the body to heal itself. The following infusion based on anti-microbial and eliminative actions is suitable for the early stages of almost any acute condition. It also provides a good basis for adaptation to individual needs.

Marigold
Thyme or Sage
Vervain   in equal parts

Fever

A fever, or raised body temperature, is a sign that the body is fighting an illness, most commonly an acute viral or bacterial infection.

An infection begins when micro-organisms have the opportunity to multiply in the body. As micro-organisms are broken down by the immune system, waste products, called pyrogens, are released into the bloodstream and raise the body's thermostat. Through the then increasing metabolism the body swiftly addresses the infective agents. As soon as the infection is resolved, the body temperature returns to normal.

A fever, therefore, is not a disease but a defence mechanism against infections. Neither are micro-organisms the cause of infections. They are merely precipitating factors whereby already weakened resistance and lowered vitality provide the fertile ground for their proliferation.

Herbal treatment of fevers aims to support the cleansing process initiated by the body and increase its overall vitality and resistance.

Plenty of liquids are essential to encourage elimination of toxins through sweating and increased urination. The use of diuretic and diaphoretic herbs encourages this process.

A time-honoured mixture which can be drunk freely consists of the following.

Elderflower
Peppermint
Yarrow   in equal parts

Add anti-microbials, especially Marigold, Garlic or Echinacea and relaxants as needed. Meadowsweet can be used if there is much muscular or joint discomfort.

The early stages of a fever are usually accompanied by loss of appetite – a way in which our body indicates that a fast is appropriate. Do not burden the body with food at this stage, even in young children, but do drink plenty of fluid to prevent dehydration.

As the fever recedes and appetite returns, eat fruits and vegetables to nourish the body while still supporting efficient elimination, especially through the bowels.

Rest in bed throughout, keep the room temperature comfortable and the air well circulated. Frequent sponging of the head or a footbath with tepid water or herbal infusions is refreshing and keeps a raised body temperature at bay. Most fevers are self-limiting with the temperature returning to normal within two days. Allow for adequate convalescence in order to regain full vitality.

Call professional help immediately if:

■ the fever is persistently over 39 °C in children or 40 °C in adults
■ there is a febrile convulsion or a history of it
■ the temperature suddenly drops and then rises again

■ the temperature drops below 35 °C together with cold, clammy
  skin and drowsiness.

Chronic conditions

Repeated or prolonged episodes of ill-health gradually corrode the
body's defences and penetrate into increasingly deeper layers
leading to progressively more deep-seated, hence chronic,
conditions. These will not only affect the functioning of our body,
but gradually damage its structure such as joints, heart, blood
vessels, lungs and affect glandular and hormonal responses, which
mediate our deeper immune processes.

A weakened immune system is characterized by:

■ slow recovery from minor infections
■ frequent and recurrent infections
■ general exhaustion and fatigue
■ the development of chronic complaints such as digestive
  problems, skin complaints, arthritis, circulatory deficiencies
■ allergies and food sensitivities.

To activate the immune system, support and tone the digestive
system, gently improve elimination through the bowels, urinary
system, lymphatics and the skin and consider the use of nervines
and adrenal tonics to improve energy levels. Allow for adequate
rest and draw on supportive measures such as meditation,
relaxation, yoga, t'ai chi, etc.

The following mixture drunk regularly over a period of time
supports effective elimination and provides nourishment with a
warming stimulating touch due to the Ginger.

Borage	
Dandelion root	
Marigold	
Nettle	
Vervain	in equal parts
with a pinch of Ginger	

In addition, consider the following:

- Evaluate your diet and lifestyle.
- Assess all stresses in your life.
- Address all infections promptly.
- Always allocate time for convalescence when unwell.

7 | THE CIRCULATORY SYSTEM

In essence the heart and the blood vessels carry all the essential nutrients to every cell in the body and remove the metabolic waste produced through the body's many actions and functions. The circulatory system, therefore, connects and affects all bodily systems and in turn is also influenced by them. If, for example, there is weakness in an organ, it may be that the organ is not sufficiently supplied with nutrients from the blood carried in the blood vessels or that metabolic waste produced by that organ is not effectively removed by the circulatory system.

Anatomy and physiology

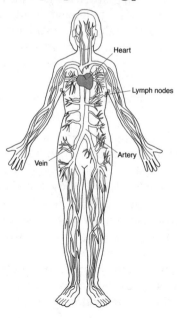

The circulatory system consists of:

- the heart
- the blood vessels
- the blood.

The heart

The heart, a muscular organ that contracts rhythmically, is the centre of the circulatory system as it forces the blood through a system of vessels. Within 24 hours the heart of an adult pumps 36,000 litres of blood through the 20,000 kilometres of blood vessels. It beats between 65 and 80 beats per minute.

The blood vessels

Arteries are blood vessels that proceed from the heart and generally (although not in the case of the pulmonary artery) carry oxygenated blood. They are hollow, elastic tubes that decrease in size as they spread through the body. The smaller arteries are called capillaries.

Veins are blood vessels that proceed towards the heart and generally (although not in the case of the pulmonary vein) carry deoxygenated blood. They are also elastic tubes, but, in addition, have valves that prevent any backflow of blood as it returns to the heart.

The blood

The blood, about 4–5 litres in the adult, is made up of four main components:

- Plasma provides the liquid base of the blood in which sugar, amino acids, mineral salts and enzymes (which may be waste or nutrients etc.) float.
- Red blood cells, erythrocytes, are the body's transporters. They carry the oxygen from the lungs to all parts of the body and collect waste products, mainly carbon dioxide, for elimination through the lungs. Haemoglobin is the oxygen-carrying pigment of the erythrocytes.
- White blood cells, leucocytes, are the protectors of the body against infections. They can ingest disease-carrying microbes and produce antibodies to neutralize them.

■ Platelets are essential to the blood for clotting or coagulation.

The circulation is divided into two main systems:

■ The general, also called systemic, circulation carries blood around the body; it includes two sub-systems: the portal circulation that conveys blood from the digestive system to the liver, and the coronary circulation that supplies the heart.

■ The pulmonary circulation carries blood to and from the lungs.

The blood is oxygenated in the lungs and flows through the pulmonary veins, the only veins carrying oxygenated blood, to the left side of the heart. From here it is pumped through the aorta, the body's longest artery, to the body and distributed throughout the network of arteries and finally capillaries. Here blood is carried right into the cells where the oxygen is needed for cell respiration.

The capillaries then join together to form increasingly larger veins which transport the deoxygenated blood from the cells to the heart. The veins empty the deoxygenated blood into the right side of the heart where it is pumped, through the pulmonary artery, to the lungs for reoxygenation as well as the release of carbon dioxide and some water. In addition to oxygen, the blood also carries nutrients. These are picked up from the food in the digestive system and the liver. In the kidneys, water and waste products carried in the blood are filtered from it and eliminated.

Herbs for the circulatory system

Heart tonics

Heart tonics are used specifically to strengthen the heart. They act by improving the contraction of the heart muscle and dilating the blood vessels of the heart circulation. Over time, the use of heart tonics will normalize the function of the heart.

Hawthorn is the most widely used heart tonic.

Peripheral vasodilators

These promote the production of prostaglandins, which relax the muscles of the blood vessels. This allows for increased circulation of the blood through the opened vessel. Vasodilation is particularly noticeable in blood vessels close to the surface of the skin as it may also increase sweating (see diaphoretics):

Garlic
Limeflower
Yarrow

Circulatory stimulants

These tend to quicken the physiological process of the circulation, hence they are often warming and stimulating:

Cinnamon
Garlic
Ginger
Rosemary

Herbs affecting the blood vessels

These herbs will help to strengthen, tone and repair damaged vessel walls and to control cholesterol levels:

Garlic
Horsechestnut
Horsetail
Lime flower
Marigold
Nettle
Rosemary

Diuretics

Diuretics will increase the flow of urine from the kidneys. At times they are called for to address water retention due to a heart weakness:

Dandelion
Horsetail
Nettle
Yarrow

Nervines

Given the prominent role stress and anxiety play in causing cardiovascular problems, the use of nervines with particular affinity for the circulation may need to be considered:

Lavender
Lemon Balm
Lime flower
Rosemary
Skullcap
Vervain

Complaints of the circulatory system

In western societies, circulatory and heart diseases contribute significantly to long-term ill-health and cause more than half of all deaths. Most health problems, including those of the circulatory system, take many years to develop and much can be done to prevent them.

The use of herbs can be no substitute for active prevention.

Prevention of circulatory disorders

■ Regular exercise is vital to keep the whole system toned and active.

■ The single most important dietary approach is to lower the intake of fats, be they saturated or unsaturated. The high salt intake in western diets is also a concern.

■ Anyone concerned about their health should stop smoking and reduce alcohol consumption to a moderate level.

■ Stress and anxiety play a prominent role in the occurrence of health problems, particularly in the cardiovascular system. Anyone prone to anxiety and tension would do well to consider their ability to deal with the stresses in their lives, and make, if necessary, lifestyle changes and learn suitable relaxation and meditation techniques.

Problems in this system can arise directly in the actions and functions of the heart, in the general blood circulation and the state of the blood vessels. In addition, water retention due to weak fluid elimination occurs commonly in prolonged circulatory disorders and needs to be considered, as does the well-being of the nervous system which so often contributes to cardiovascular problems. (Weaknesses caused by circulatory disorders, but manifesting in other bodily systems as well as ill-health in other systems and other influences on the circulatory system have to be excluded here.)

While herbal medicine has much to offer in the treatment of cardiovascular problems, it is essential that all serious conditions should be attended by a medical practitioner.

Weakness of the heart

Most circulatory conditions benefit from direct attention to the functions of the heart.

Hawthorn is the most outstanding normalizer of heart function, with an overall toning and strengthening effect. It is suitable for people with high or low blood pressure as it will relax or stimulate the heart according to need.

I tend to make use of the different energy of the tops (the flowers and leaves) and the berries. The tops with their light, uplifting spring energy are suitable for people who need nourishing and boosting of the heart and circulatory energy, whereas the berries have an affinity with a calm and relaxing autumn energy. I use them for people who are in need of relaxing and focusing on themselves.

Preparations of Hawthorn can be taken long term as a tonic for heart function.

Palpitations

Palpitations indicate an awareness of the heartbeat. Common manifestations are:

- The heartbeat may suddenly pound and increase.
- Episodes may last from a few minutes to several hours.
- Palpitations may be caused by anxiety, fear, exercise, smoking, alcohol and excessive coffee consumption.
- Mostly palpitations are not an indication of disease but may be linked to anaemia and thyroid disorders and should always be taken seriously.

For isolated palpitations the following tea is soothing, calming and reassuring.

> Skullcap
> Lemon Balm   in equal parts
>
> If there is any sign of increased blood pressure, add Hawthorn.

High blood pressure

The causes of high blood pressure fall into two groups:

- Well-defined physical problems account for about 10% of cases of high blood pressure. They will not be discussed here.
- In contrast, essential hypertension is a common problem in western societies. It is said to occur without a clear cause but a predisposing family history is often found as is an inappropriate diet, lack of exercise and long-term stress (see above). In this situation, herbs have a significant role to play.

Common symptoms

- headache, especially in the morning
- dizziness and visual disturbances
- ringing in the ears
- fatigue and inability to concentrate
- breathlessness and angina-like pains.

In addition to strengthening the heart with Hawthorn, the peripheral circulation can be improved with vasodilators. Given the predominance of emotional and physical tension an appropriate nervine should be added to any mixture.

Two basic effective mixtures, that can be adapted to individual requirements are:

■ for a low-energy person:

Hawthorn tops	
Yarrow	
Vervain	in equal parts
a pinch of Ginger	

■ for a high-energy, stressed person:

Hawthorn berries	
Lemon Balm	
Limeflower	in equal parts

For dietary and lifestyle suggestions see above.

Low blood pressure

While most of us are aware of the dangers of high blood pressure, low blood pressure can just as deeply affect our well-being. It is usually caused by organic disease and manifests with:

■ dizziness and fainting
■ headaches, fatigue and inability to concentrate
■ increasing exhaustion and debility.

In addition to treating the underlying cause, good food, gentle exercise and regular rest are important.

A gently warming and energising mixture consists of:

Ginger	
Hawthorn tops	
Rosemary	in equal parts
Nettle with its nourishing action can also be added.	

Arteriosclerosis

This is a generic term for a number of diseases in which the arterial wall becomes thickened, hardened and loses elasticity.

In the early stages, mineral deposits attach themselves along the artery and restrict the flow of blood to the body cells. Later in the process, cholesterol and fatty deposits, called atheroma, build up. They can be found in the aorta and the arteries of the brain and heart. An atheroma may block an artery in itself or precipitate a clot or embolism. It may travel to a smaller artery where it can become lodged and cause serious damage and even death.

Arteriosclerosis can be the forerunner of degenerative heart and kidney disease and is often associated with high blood pressure.

Minor symptoms

■ cold hands and feet
■ possibly dizziness and headaches
■ breathlessness and fatigue.

The causes of arteriosclerosis are typically long-term stress and tension, a sedentary lifestyle with a diet high in fat, salt, alcohol and smoking. Hereditary weakness of the blood vessels may also contribute as can the toxic effects of environmental poisons.

In addition to lifestyle and dietary changes (see above), herbs have a major role to play in addressing the problem.

Garlic is well known to help reduce cholesterol levels and reverse any plaque formation that has already started. Buckwheat, Alfalfa, Artichoke and Linseed act similarly and, like Garlic, need to be used on a regular basis.

Limeflowers specific for protecting and repairing arteries and combines well with Marigold for healing and strengthening of the bloodvessels and Nettle for the reduction of cholesterol levels. As any damage to blood vessels increases the workload of the heart, Hawthorn should be added.

A pleasant-tasting mixture which can be used long term is the following:

Hawthorn	1 part
Limeflower	2 parts
Marigold	1 part
Nettle	1 part
Yarrow	1 part

Varicose veins

Varicose veins are dilated, swollen and twisted veins, often due to valve weakness, which allows for backflow of blood, or increased blood pressure.

Distended veins can be found anywhere in the body. Common sites are in the lower legs, around the anus, where they are called haemorrhoids or piles and around the testicles, where they are called varicoceles.

Symptoms in the legs include:

■ visible veins, which may or may not be painful

■ aching legs

■ tingling and increased heat in the legs.

Symptoms often can be relieved by raising and resting the legs; they should not be massaged.

Pregnancy may lead to or aggravate varicose veins or piles; any existing ones may be worse during menstruation.

Horsechestnut protects and tones veins and can be combined with herbs to stimulate the peripheral circulation and support the heart.

The following mixture can be taken long term:

Hawthorn	
Horsechestnut	
Yarrow	in equal parts
with a pinch of Ginger	

> If there is much water retention around the ankles, Dandelion
> herb is an effective diuretic and may need to be added until
> swellings reduce.

Good pelvic circulation needs to be ensured by taking regular
exercise, wearing loose clothes and avoiding sitting cross-legged.
Constipation can also impair the circulation to the legs and needs to
be addressed, if an issue.

Iron-deficiency anaemia

This is characterized by a reduction in the haemoglobin levels of
the blood leading to progressive oxygen starvation of all tissues.

This can give rise to the following symptoms:

- constant tiredness and lethargy
- dizziness and headaches
- breathlessness and palpitations, especially on exercise
- indigestion
- irritability, mood swings and depression.

Usually iron-deficiency anaemia develops gradually over a period
of time; it often goes undetected until a range of symptoms alerts to
the possibility. About 15% of women are anaemic.

Common causes are:

- heavy menstrual bleeding
- pregnancy
- poor diet and mineral deficiencies
- unknown blood loss e.g. from haemorrhoids or gastric ulcers
- worms
- rheumatoid arthritis
- lack of hydrochloric acid in the stomach.

Bitter herbs stimulate the absorption of vital nutrients from the
digestive system and increase appetite. A number of herbs are
especially rich in iron such as Nettle, Horsetail and Comfrey and as
many as possible should be used.

A basic mixture contains:

Dandelion root	
Horsetail	
Nettle	in equal parts

Make sure your diet is rich in iron-containing foods such as pulses, nuts, watercress, Alfalfa, beetroot, dark green vegetables, apricots. Eat plenty of fresh fruit and vegetables as Vitamin C enhances iron absorption and sip a little cider vinegar in water before meals to increase stomach acidity.

Avoid the following as they limit iron absorption:

■ antacids and tetracyclines
■ chocolate, coffee, tea, especially with meals
■ wheat bran and excessive amounts of wholemeal bread.

The Lymphatic System

The lymphatic system is a secondary circulation intertwined with the blood circulation assisting particularly the veins in recovering the body's tissue fluids and returning them to the heart. Its function is to give nourishment to body cells and in return remove their wasteproducts and together with the immune system, build up resistance against infections.

The basic component of the lymphatic system is the **lymph**, a pale yellow fluid similar to the fluid which oozes from a cut when bleeding stops.

Lymph is drained by small lymphatic vessels which gradually increase in size as they move lymph towards the heart. Similar to veins, larger lymph vessels are supplied with valves. Interspersed along the route to the heart are **lymph nodes**, which vary in size from pin-heads to nuts. Their function is to filter the lymph of microbial substances and therefore help to prevent the spread of infections into the bloodstream. Lymphocytes, white bloodcells suspended in the lymphatic fluid and one of the principal cells of the immune system, are added to the lymph fluid to support this action. It is the superficial lymph nodes such as at the neck, under the arms or in the groin, and the tonsils, which may enlarge when an infection is present in the body and actively addressed by the immune system. Eventually, all lymph fluid passes into the two main lymphatic vessels, the thoracic and lymphatic ducts at the neck. These interconnect with the bloodstream at the base of the neck where the lymph system becomes again part of the general blood circulation.

Herbs for the lymphatic system

These are called **alteratives**; they favourably change the blood and lymph to detoxify and renew body tissues. In older herbal books they are often referred to as blood-cleansers.

Cleavers	Marigold
Echinacea	Red Clover

Complaints of the lymphatic system

As the lymphatic system also builds up immunity against infections, its role in holistic health is of considerable and far-reaching importance.

Poor lymphatic drainage and chronically enlarged lymph nodes can prevent effective waste elimination, as the lymphatic fluid then becomes overburdened by excess toxins and metabolic waste products. Thus, the ground may be prepared for long-term, chronic disorders.

Alteratives can be added in any situation where the lymphatic system needs support such as chronic catarrh, tonsillitis and glandular fever.

A useful base mixture to support the system whenever a problem arises is:

Cleavers	2 parts
Marigold	1 part

In conjunction with herbs, a cleansing regime is also usually needed. A fruit and vegetable based diet is especially effective as it will give the body a break from difficult to process or inappropriate foods such as excessive quantities of cow's milk, dairy produce, red meats, fatty foods, refined carbohydrates and sugars. Alcohol, tea and coffee consumption should be avoided and plenty of water and detoxifying herbal teas such as Nettle or Dandelion leaf should be drunk instead.

8 | THE RESPIRATORY SYSTEM

The continuous, often unconscious ebb and flow of our breath draws life energy into our being. The open flow of breathing is one of the keys not only to our health but also to our experience of life, as each breath we take connects us to our inner and outer environments. It is therefore no surprise that during times past and present as well as in diverse cultures the role of breath is central to concepts of the body and well-being, and many spiritual practices build on the dynamic and vitality of breathing.

Through inhalation the body absorbs from the atmosphere the oxygen needed by every cell in the body to utilize the energy provided by the nutrients of our food. Exhalation discharges waste from the metabolism of our body in the form of carbon dioxide. This in turn nourishes plant life which depends on it for its own life cycles.

Normal function of all body cells is maintained by the adequate supply of nutrients and oxygen throughout the blood and efficient elimination of waste. To ensure sufficient oxygen is supplied, we need to breathe adequately, take regular exercise and breathe fresh air. The best prevention of respiratory disease is clean air. The less polluted the atmosphere we breathe in, the less pollution and waste our bodies will have to cope with.

Anatomy and physiology

The respiratory system is responsible for taking in oxygen and giving off carbon dioxide and some water.

Each minute an adults breathes in and out approximately 16 times; this is increased considerably when taking exercise.

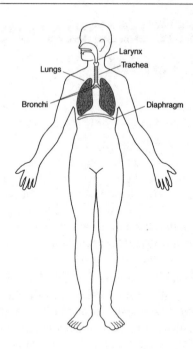

The respiratory system is divided into:

■ upper respiratory tract which includes:

- nose
- mouth
- throat
- larynx (voicebox)
- sinus cavities in the head

■ lower respiratory tract, which includes:

- trachea (windpipe)
- bronchi
- lungs
- diaphragm.

The respiratory system is lined throughout with mucous membranes. In order to avoid any drying out of the membranes, a small amount of mucus is continuously produced.

Air taken in through the nose and to a lesser extent the mouth is filtered and warmed before passing into the bronchi and from there to the lungs.

Each bronchus is divided into smaller and smaller branches, the bronchioles, which terminate in the alveoli, little air sacs. These are made of elastic tissue, so that they expand when filled with air. It is between the alveoli and the surrounding network of capillaries that the exchange of oxygen and carbon dioxide takes place. Here, oxygen passes into the bloodstream and is carried by the haemoglobin part of the blood to all the cells of the body. At the same time the blood releases carbon dioxide from cell metabolism into the alveoli from where it is expelled into the atmosphere when breathing out.

The lungs are inert organs and cannot work by themselves. The diaphragm, a muscular wall, and the muscles of the ribcage enable the lungs to function.

On breathing in, the muscles between the ribs contract; the contraction lifts the ribcage upwards and outwards depressing the diaphragm. This allows the air to rush into the lungs and fill the space created by the change in atmospheric pressure. Breathing out relaxes the muscles between the ribs and the diaphragm. The relaxation increases atmospheric pressure and deflates the lungs. Carbon dioxide and water are therefore released into the air.

Herbs for the respiratory system

Anti-catarrhals

These herbs reduce the production of mucus and help to remove any excess phlegm. They are often aromatic and astringent and also offer protection to the mucous membranes:

Elderflower
Mullein
Peppermint
Ribwort
Sage
Yarrow

Anti-microbials and antiseptics

These help the body to destroy or resist micro-organisms, prevent infection and reduce their impact:

Cinnamon	Liquorice	Sage
Echinacea	Peppermint	Thyme
Garlic	Ribwort	
Lavender	Rosemary	

Alteratives

Alteratives help to detoxify the blood and lymphatic system; they are often called for in conditions of excess mucus and with frequent infection:

Cleavers	Marigold
Echinacea	Nettle

Demulcents

These moisturize, soothe and protect irritated respiratory membranes and are often helpful to ease dry coughs:

Comfrey	Marshmallow
Liquorice	Mullein

Diaphoretics

Diaphoretics promote sweating and the elimination of toxins through the skin; they may be warming or cooling:

Elderflower	Peppermint
Ginger	Vervain
Lemon Balm	Yarrow
Limeflower	

Anti-spasmodics

These prevent and relieve muscular spasms such as in unproductive coughs:

Chamomile	Liquorice	Mullein
Cramp Bark	Lemon Balm	Red Clover
Fennel	Limeflower	Vervain

Expectorants

Expectorants help to expel excess mucus from the lungs, through either soothing or irritating actions:

Fennel	Liquorice	Red Clover
Garlic	Marshmallow	Ribwort
Ginger	Mullein	Thyme

Complaints of the upper respiratory system

Respiratory problems can originate in the respiratory system itself, as it is open to airborne infections. But the lungs, together with the digestive system, the urinary system and the skin are also pathways for excretion of toxins.

Excess toxins in the body can place an extra burden on the respiratory system, just as a respiratory problem can add pressure to other organs and systems of elimination.

As we shall see, this dynamic is taken into account in holistic treatment.

The most common complaints in the upper respiratory system result from problems with the mucous membranes that line the nose, mouth, throat and sinuses. Problems in this area usually lead to catarrh and vulnerability to infection. Treatment will therefore mostly focus on restoring mucus and mucous membrane conditions and decongesting respiratory passages.

Catarrh

A small amount of mucus is continuously produced by the upper respiratory system to provide the moisture needed by the mucous membranes. The excessive stimulation of this natural production of mucus known as catarrh can be due to various factors. Most commonly it is the result of:

- internal accumulation of toxins from an inappropriate diet
- allergies (hay fever, asthma)
- external pollutants (dust, exhaust fumes and cigarette smoke)
- acute or chronic infections.

In conditions associated with catarrh, the body uses the excess mucus as a mechanism to protect mucous membranes and to facilitate waste removal not effectively eliminated elsewhere.

To address catarrh effectively, one's diet needs to be assessed and a low mucus-forming diet should be followed (see below).

The following herbs may be helpful to tone mucous membranes, dry up excessive secretions and support the body as a whole to remove toxins through the lymphatic system:

> Cleavers
> Elderflower
> Peppermint   in equal parts
>
> In addition, steam inhalation with Chamomile or Chamomile and Peppermint helps to relieve nasal congestion.

In hay fever a combination of:

> Chamomile
> Elderflower
> Nettle   in equal parts

may be considered. Local honey may also help to reduce allegic responses.

Low mucus-forming diet

A low mucus-forming diet focuses on limiting the intake of foods that feed the mucus-forming mechanisms of the body. Prime dietary sources of mucus-producing foods are cow's milk products such as milk, cheese, yoghurt and carbohydrates, especially when refined.

Sensitivity or allergy to dairy products (sometimes including goat's milk) can cause persistent catarrh and give rise to frequent infections. Should you be prone to coughs and colds, it is probably best to avoid it during the winter months. Children who frequently suffer from upper respiratory tract infections, glue ear or coughs are likely to have a milk intolerance and would benefit greatly to have it removed *completely* from their diet.

As mucus is a naturally occurring body carbohydrate, to restrict dietary carbohydrate intake, particularly the gluten-rich grains such as wheat, barley, rye and oat as well as sugar is also advisable.

If the problem is severe or prolonged, bananas, rich in mucus, and starchy root vegetables such as potatoes and swede should also be limited. The irritation to mucous membranes caused by peanuts often compounds the formation of excess mucus and it is usually helpful to exclude them from the diet.

These foods should be replaced with plenty of fresh fruit, fruit juices, salads, vegetables and pulses.

To encourage elimination through the kidneys and bowels, plenty of fluids should be drunk and, if needed, supported with Burdock and Dandelion root, Celery seed and Nettle. In addition, hot (fresh) lemon and honey drinks are helpful to loosen and break down any excess mucus.

Common cold

The cause of the common cold is an acute viral infection with inflammation affecting especially the upper respiratory system.

A cold begins usually with:

- sore throat
- discomfort in the nose, followed by sneezing
- feeling 'under the weather'
- a profusely runny nose with watery discharge.

Gradually the nasal discharge becomes more solid and resembles severe catarrh and, typically there is no fever.

Symptoms should clear up within 4–10 days, although occasionally a cough may develop and bacterial complications can cause sinusitis and ear infections.

The first step in the treatment of the common cold is to follow a low mucus-forming diet. If you are prone to colds, it may be wise to restrict mucus-forming foods during the winter months. At the same time your body will need extra vitamin C to fight the infection and plenty of fresh fruit and fruit juices should be part of your diet.

A time-honoured mixture, and one of my favourites, is:

> Elderflower
> Peppermint
> Yarrow   in equal parts
>
> Drink 4–6 cups daily until symptoms subside.
>
> For extra vitamin C, Rosehip could be added.
>
> For a more warming tea, a pinch of dried Ginger or some Cinnamon bark would be a good complement.

Sinusitis

This condition is an infection of the sinus cavities in the head commonly caused by streptococcal infection.

Acute sinusitis

Acute sinusitis can cause:

- pain and swelling in the face, around the nose, cheeks, eyes and forehead
- headaches
- toothache.

The following mixture is effective in the acute phase:

> Echinacea
> Elderflower
> Thyme or Peppermint   in equal parts
>
> The addition of Marshmallow or Ribwort is useful to soothe inflamed membranes, if there is much soreness and pain. A simple Ginger compress over the cheeks and forehead may also provide much relief, as may regular steam inhalations.

Chronic sinusitis

Acute infection can lead to a chronic, often persistent, condition:

■ The sinus cavities become inflamed and congested with mucus, possibly blocking the passages to the nose.
■ The mucus may be purulent.
■ There may be loss of sense of smell.

Guidelines for catarrh should be followed, especially a low mucus-forming diet with plenty of fresh fruit and garlic.

To help decongest and soothe irritated sinuses in the chronic conditions, adjust your diet and regularly drink:

Elderflower	
Peppermint	
Ribwort	in equal parts

Ear infection

Infections of the ear are commonly caused by streptococci and spread from the nose and throat via the Eustachian tubes to the middle ear.

First signs of an acute earache are:

■ intense pain
■ deafness in the affected ear
■ a fever.

Address all ear complaints promptly, especially in children; if there is a discharge from the ear, seek professional advice immediately.

Echinacea	
Elderflower	
Mullein or Ribwort	
St John's Wort	in equal parts

If there is a raised temperature, add Peppermint to the mixture.

Drunk throughout the day this will help to address the infection, reduce the catarrhal build-up and generally relax.

Provided there is no pus in the ear, a few drops of warmed infused Mullein oil, St John's Wort oil or Garlic oil (from a pricked capsule) can be dropped into the ear or, instead, rubbed behind it. Regular steam inhalation loosens the mucus and eases the infection; a warm water bottle against the affected ear provides much relief, but do not lie on the infected side as the mucus then cannot drain out of the ear.

Otherwise follow guidelines for catarrh.

Sore throat

The throat may be affected by a number of problems involving the upper and lower respiratory tract. These may take the form of infections of the nose, sinuses, throat, larynx, tonsils or the lungs. In addition, the voice and its use in communication and creative expression is associated in holistic approaches to health with the throat area. If there is any unexpressed emotion or inhibited creativity, these may cause problems in this area such as loss of voice, hoarseness, chronic inflammation etc. Therefore the causes need to be looked for in order for any problems to be addressed effectively.

A common cause of transient sore throat, noticeable on waking in the morning, is central heating. The low air humidity causes a drying of the mucous membranes which in turn increases nasal mucus. The resultant nasal congestion causes mouth breathing and subsequent irritation of the mucous membranes in the mouth and throat, which we experience as a sore throat. This can easily be remedied by ensuring circulation of fresh air throughout the night and placing vaporizers or bowls of water on the radiators.

Throat infections

This type of infection can be either bacterial or viral in origin.

A bacterial infection is likely to be caused by the streptococcal bacterium and leads to:

■ a severe sore throat

■ swollen glands (to check for swollen glands gently run your
  fingers from the ears down to below the jaw and chin)

■ general malaise with or without a raised temperature.

A viral infection leads to:

■ a sore throat

■ a runny nose or nasal congestion

■ weepy eyes

■ a slight cough.

Throat swabs to be taken for culture can confirm the origin
although in most cases the above guidelines are likely to be
sufficient.

For sore throats in general, a gargle with *Red* or *Garden Sage* with
a little honey, every hour or two is a very effective antiseptic; if
there is much dryness, the addition of *Marshmallow* or *Ribwort* is
soothing and protective to the delicate membranes. The same tea
should also be drunk several times a day to support the immune
system.

If the tonsils (lymphatic tissue at either side of the throat), the
adenoids (lymphatic tissue at the back of the nose) or any other
lymph glands in the neck are swollen, it is an indication that the
lymphatic system is fulfilling its role in protecting the body.

To support the lymphatic system in its protecting and cleansing
work, alterative herbs should be considered.

These pleasant-tasting mixtures combine antiseptic, soothing and
cleansing actions:

Marigold or	Cleavers	
Ribwort	Marshmallow	
Sage	Thyme	in equal parts

Liquorice and spices such as Cinnamon or Ginger could be
added to taste and to increase the warming qualities of the
infusion.

Tonsillitis

The inflammation of the tonsils (tonsillitis) demonstrates that the glands are fulfilling their role in protecting the body against micro-organisms.The tonsils together with the adenoids provide a barrier against pollution and infections entering the body through the mouth and the nose. At the same time, like other lymphatic tissue in the body, they act as screens for poisons in the bloodstream, in the case of tonsillitis especially those draining from the nose and sinuses. Because of their supporting role, tonsils should not be removed surgically unless there are very good reasons to do so.

Tonsillitis may be acute or chronic in response to a viral or bacterial infection.

Acute tonsillitis

- The tonsils become swollen, inflamed and painful.
- There is marked difficulty in swallowing.
- Viral tonsillitis is often preceded by low vitality and a general catarrhal respiratory problem such as a cold or flu of viral origin.
- Bacterial tonsillitis tends to start suddenly with a very painful sore throat (see above), swollen neck glands and is often accompanied by a fever.

Treatment aims at supporting the body and aiding the glands in their work. At the appearance of the first symptoms frequent hot infusions are helpful.

Elderflower
Marigold
Ribwort
Sage   in equal parts

A Red Sage gargle and inhalations with Chamomile, Peppermint, Thyme or Lavender complement the infusion very well.

A low-mucus diet should be followed to ease the load on the lymphatic system with plenty of fresh fruit, juices, fresh lemon and honey drinks and vegetable soups.

Chronic tonsillitis

This condition is indicated by:

■ frequent bouts of acute tonsillitis
■ the tonsils remain swollen and at times inflamed and painful in between times.

This state is often the result of the overuse of antibiotics to treat acute infections. It may also be an indication that toxins are continously drained from nasal catarrh, congested ears etc. due to, for example, an allegic response to milk products and the resultant excessive production of mucus.

Treatment essentially follows the suggestions for acute tonsillitis, with particular emphasis on support for the lymphatic system, through the inclusion of, for example, Cleavers in any mixture and the adherence to a low mucus-forming diet.

Laryngitis

Infections from the mouth, nose or throat can spread to the larynx causing inflammation and infection. Laryngitis is therefore often associated with flu or colds, tonsillitis and bronchitis.

Acute laryngitis

■ The larynx feels sore.
■ The voice may be absent or hoarse.
■ There is pain on talking.

While acute laryngitis is mostly self-limiting if the voice is rested, suggestions for tonsillitis are also applicable. Acute laryngitis, especially in children, should not be neglected as it can lead to more serious respiratory problems.

Chronic laryngitis

This is commonly due to the malfunction of the vocal cords mainly from stress, overuse of the voice, smoking and polyps on the vocal cords.

It is characterized by:

■ hoarseness
■ pain on speaking
■ loss of voice.

Soothing and calming infusions, gargles and inhalations (see tonsillitis) are all helpful. If the condition persists, consult a medical practitioner.

Complaints of the lower respiratory system

Diseases of the lower respiratory system abound and are often confusing in the details of their signs and symptoms. On closer inspection, these diseases can be seen as broadly falling into two categories.

First, problems with the mucous membranes that line bronchi, bronchioles and lungs can lead to congestion of the lungs and subsequent vulnerability to infections. Each part of the lower respiratory system can develop inflammations and infections. Similarities with the upper respiratory system will be noticeable.

The second significant type of respiratory problems are associated with the muscles of the bronchi, lungs and ribcage that control the airflow within the lungs and in and out of them. As a result of complex interactions between a number of different factors ranging from possible allergies to the state of the nervous system, muscle spasms can severely limit lung function.

Coughs

A cough is the body's protective reflex to clear the throat and bronchi of any obstruction and irritation. This can be food or drink that has been swallowed the wrong way, environmental irritants such as fumes, cigarette smoke or inflammation and infection in any part of the lower respiratory system causing irritation and increased mucus in the respiratory passages.

Suppression of coughs is not helpful as the cough is a natural, protective response to a problem and not its cause.

Coughs fall into two categories and herbal treatment depends on the type of cough and any surrounding circumstances.

However, as with catarrh in the upper respiratory system, all coughs and chest infections call for a low mucus-forming diet (for details see under Catarrh). A cough syrup is often the most appropriate preparation for coughs, although the following suggestions for infusion are nevertheless effective.

Dry cough

Dry, irritating and at times hacking coughs are caused by irritation in the throat and lungs due to:

- environmental irritants such as a dry atmosphere, chemicals, fumes and cigarette smoke
- a foreign body in the respiratory passages
- anxiety and stress
- early viral or bacterial infection in the lower respiratory system, such as bronchitis
- spread of infections from the ears, sinuses and the tonsils.

In the treatment of dry, irritating coughs the aim is to soothe and protect mucous membranes as well as to loosen the accumulating mucus with demulcents.

In addition, respiratory relaxants may be needed to ease tension and allow the flow of mucus to take place. Choose any of the aromatic herbs as they are also antiseptic.

Mullein works well in dry coughs in the following combination:

Mullein	2 parts
Ribwort or Liquorice	1 part

Add Lavender or Vervain if there is much tension in the muscles, headache or a fever.

I also add Vervain for children if they are irritable, whingey and restless.

Regular steam inhalations offer much relief as does the use of an antiseptic and relaxing chest balm.

Productive cough

This type of cough is likely to be caused by the lungs producing excess mucus. This can be due to:

■ an infection such as a cold, flu or bronchitis

■ an allergy as in asthma

■ congestion due to the accumulation of toxic waste from elsewhere in the body, inadequate diet and lifestyle

■ any form of lowered vitality which provides an ideal breeding ground for subsequent infection and irritation.

Treatment of productive coughs aims to encourage the loosening and the expectoration of excessive mucus, be it due to overproduction or inadequate excretion.

Respiratory stimulants are called for in this situation as they stimulate the nerves and muscles of the respiratory system and trigger the cough reflex.

I have found the infusion combining soothing, stimulating and antiseptic properties, very helpful.

Mullein
Ribwort
Thyme   in equal parts

This combination works well with some Ginger and Garlic for added warmth and a dispersing stimulus.

If your problem is more chronic, it may be related to a general overload of toxins. Consider possible allergies, bowel function and urinary output. If appropriate, support all eliminative functions (see catarrh).

Asthma

The most common respiratory problem characterized by spasms in the respiratory passages is asthma.

Asthma is caused by spasmodic contraction of the bronchi and bronchioles following respiratory infections, emotional tension, exercise and allergies. The obstruction of the airways leads to difficulties with breathing, especially breathing out, which produces a typical wheezing or whistling sound.

Common symptoms of an acute asthma attack are:

■ acute breathlessness
■ difficulty breathing out
■ wheezing
■ coughing
■ sense of chest constriction.

In between attacks people tend to be well, although a continous wheeziness may remain. Asthma in general is related to low vitality, respiratory weakness, allergies and emotional stresses. In some cases there is an inherited disposition whereby asthma and also eczema and hay fever runs in the family. Many asthmatics have environmental or food allergies where cow's milk produce, wheat, eggs and artificial food additives are common food allergens and pollen, dust, animal furs and fumes are frequent environmental triggers. In others, tension, anxiety, hyperactivity or physical exertion can cause constriction of the airways and trigger an attack. Any respiratory infection and the concomitant irritation and excess mucus can lead to bronchial spasms and an asthma attack.

As asthma can be due to a combination of any of these factors, it is important to address this problem holistically and identify all contributing aspects. Only general suggestions can be offered here.

Herbs to soothe and relax the irritated airways, such as Mullein and Ribwort, can be combined with expectorants like Thyme. To support the nervous system Vervain or Skullcap make helpful additions, as does Liquorice to aid the long-term health of the adrenal glands and overall immunity. If the asthma particularly affects the circulation and the heart, Hawthorn or Limeflower could be considered. All respiratory infections should be treated promptly in order to avoid low general well-being and vitality. As allergies play such an important part in asthma, careful attention should be paid to an appropriate, mostly low mucus-forming diet.

9 | THE DIGESTIVE SYSTEM

The digestive system is concerned with the breakdown, digestion and assimilation of food and the elimination of waste products resulting from this process. It transforms, particularly in conjunction with the respiratory system, foods into available energies necessary for the activities of our daily living as well as the requirements of the body's biochemical processes such as growth, repair and the production of heat. The dual aspect of openness to the outer world and traversing through our inner body makes the digestive system at the same time one of the most significant interfaces between our inner and outer environments.

Our health and vitality depend to a large degree on how well our digestive system functions in utilizing the nutrients supplied by our food for our body. Increasingly, we realize that health depends not only on what we eat but equally on how effectively our digestive system absorbs and assimilates the food eaten and eliminates any waste. To approach the understanding of digestive health in a holistic way, the complexity of the entire process needs to be appreciated.

Anatomy and physiology

The digestive tract consists of:
- the mouth
- the pharynx
- oesophagus
- stomach
- small intestines
- large intestines
- the rectum
- the anus.

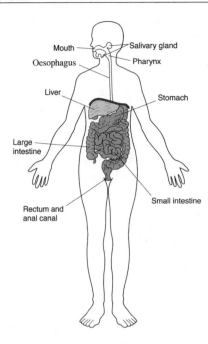

Associated with it are the accessory organs:
- the tongue
- teeth
- salivary glands
- liver and gall bladder
- pancreas.

The digestive process begins in the mouth where the teeth break down food through chewing while it is softened and partly digested by salivary secretions. The tongue helps in the mechanical processing of food and pushes the food into the pharynx during swallowing. The oesophagus then moves the ball-shaped food by means of muscular contractions (peristalsis) into the stomach. Here it is further mechanically broken down and through digestive juices chemically digested. The stomach contents then pass into the intricately coiled small intestines for further mechanical processing and mixing with more digestive enzymes. Liver-produced bile, stored in the gall bladder, is released into the duodenum (small intestine) as are digestive enzymes, including insulin from the pancreas. At this point most of the nutrients are sufficiently small in size and converted into simpler substances in order to be absorbed through the wall of the digestive tract into the bloodstream.

The large intestine is mostly concerned with the absorption of water, minerals and some vitamins. The remaining parts of digested food, the faeces, are moved by muscular contraction through the rectum and anus to be eliminated.

Nutrients absorbed throughout the digestive tract into the bloodstream are transported to the liver for processing and distribution to the body's cells.

In addition to the physiological factors outlined, the autonomic nervous system plays an integral part in digestive health. The nervous system contributes to the regulation of blood circulation, digestive secretions and peristaltic movements of the intestines. Strong emotions and any form of stress can have an immediate effect on the digestive system by either increasing or decreasing its finely tuned activities. Many experience either overactive or sluggish bowel movements as a result of anxiety and the concomitant changes in digestive enzyme production and peristaltic movements. To address digestive health holistically, any emotional influences and the interaction between the digestive system and the nervous system need to be fully appreciated. In addition, a diet suited to a person's needs, but generally rich in fresh, unprocessed foods with plenty of nuts, seeds, wholemeal grains, fruits and vegetables, and a generous fluid intake, is fundamental to both digestive health and general well-being.

Herbs for the digestive system

Demulcents

These can soothe and protect irritated and inflamed mucous membranes of the digestive system (see also astringents):

Comfrey	Meadowsweet
Liquorice	Oat
Marshmallow	Ribwort

Astringents

Due to their binding action on mucous membranes, astringents reduce secretions in the digestive tract and offer protection in inflamed conditions (see also demulcents):

Agrimony	Raspberry leaf
Meadowsweet	Ribwort
Nettle	

Bitters

Bitters are herbs that promote the stimulation of digestive secretions ranging from the stimulation of saliva to the increased production and flow of bile in the liver. Most are mildly laxative.

Many herbs are only slightly bitter, in addition to other more prominent actions, and others are intensely so. The following bitters are of the middle range and are often called for in holistic treatment:

Agrimony	Rosemary
Chamomile	Vervain
Dandelion root	

Carminatives

These are often aromatic herbs and spices which relax the muscles of the digestive system. This in turn reduces excess gas, eases peristalsis and improves bowel function:

Chamomile	Fennel
Celery	Peppermint
Cinnamon	

Anti-spasmodics

These relieve muscular tension, spasms and mild pain in the digestive system:

Chamomile	Peppermint
Cinnamon	Skullcap
Cramp Bark	Vervain
Lemon Balm	

Anti-microbials

These may be called for as a result of an infection giving rise to digestive problems. A weakened or overloaded digestion can also result in digestive infections:

Chamomile	Marigold
Cinnamon	Peppermint
Echinacea	Thyme

Nervines

Nervines ease emotional tension manifesting in the functioning of the digestive system:

Chamomile	Rosemary
Lavender	Skullcap
Lemon Balm	Vervain

Complaints of the digestive system

Digestive health depends on the intricate interplay of four factors in particular:

■ the integrity of the mucous membranes, which line the entire gut wall

■ the continuous flow of digestive secretions

■ regular peristaltic movements (wave-like muscular contractions of the gut wall)

■ a person's overall emotional well-being.

Many digestive complaints can be prevented by adhering to some simple guidelines that help to avoid functional problems in the digestive tract, especially the stomach, which are often the forerunners of more serious disturbances.

Our body, including the digestive system, functions according to its own innate rhythm. Yet our eating habits are increasingly determined by the demands of a pressurized lifestyle. This can lead to eating while attending to other matters, if not the outright skipping of meals, fast eating and overeating. Irregular eating disturbs the rhythm of the digestive system while fast eating and overeating burdens the digestion with an excessive and/or badly prepared load, which reduces digestive efficiency. In addition, stress, anxiety and time pressures are frequent characteristics of a modern lifestyle that negatively affect the functioning of the digestive system and the body overall. This can be exacerbated by a high intake of coffee, tea, alcohol, sugars, cigarettes and refined foods, again influencing and disturbing the digestive rhythm. Food sensitivities may also cause impaired digestive health and all foods causing problems should be avoided.

Awareness of these factors and a willingness to adapt one's diet and lifestyle accordingly will contribute significantly to the prevention of more deep-seated digestive problems.

Most digestive complaints have one or more symptoms in common and it is useful to review these together, always bearing in mind that they are not causes but manifestations of an underlying problem. It is the underlying problem that requires our holistic attention.

Loss of appetite

This is often the first indicator of digestive problems as it frees the system to deal with any upset rather than process foods. Long-term reduced appetite such as during the recovery phase from respiratory infections or chronic ill-health can be improved with the use of bitter herbs.

Diarrhoea

Diarrhoea is often the main symptom of acute digestive infection such as food poisoning, but can also be due to short- or long-term anxiety and stress causing irritation and inflammation of the gut walls and overactivity in the flow of secretions. However, symptoms of acute diarrhoea should not be suppressed as it helps to clear digestive toxins; the accompanying discomfort can be relieved with soothing, mildly astringent herbs. Generally, all carminative and anti-spasmodic herbs are suitable.

A reliable base mixture which can be adjusted to suit your needs is:

Chamomile
Meadowsweet   in equal parts

Add Lavender or Lemon Balm if there is involvement of the
nervous system; if you suspect an infection, add Echinacea or
Garlic.

Ensure good fluid intake to avoid dehydration, eat small amounts
of live yoghurt once on the way to recovery to help rebalance the
gut bacteria.

Chronic diarrhoea requires professional attention as does acute
diarrhoea in babies and young children if it lasts for more than 6
hours.

Vomiting

Like diarrhoea, vomiting is a natural response to clear toxins or
irritants from the digestive tract. The following mixture will help
settle the stomach:

Chamomile
Lemon Balm
Peppermint   in equal parts

Add Echinacea or Garlic if required.

Ensure good fluid intake to avoid dehydration. Once the stomach is
settled, eat some live yogurt to rebalance gut bacteria.

Note: If vomiting lasts for more than 24 hours, 6 hours in babies
and young children, seek professional help promptly.

Constipation

This is commonly due to a sedentary lifestyle, a diet low in fibres
and roughage, lack of fluid or emotional tension. Constipation due
to liver problems or any blockage in the intestines requires
professional attention. Regular exercise, changes in diet and plenty
of fluid can resolve many a constipation. At times herbs will also

be needed to improve the flow of gastric secretions and help retrain the muscle tone of the gut.

A pleasant-tasting and effective mixture can be prepared by using:

Burdock root	
Dandelion root	
Fennel	in equal parts

Foods such as dried prunes, rhubarb and figs and liquorice can be eaten to complement this. Fresh garlic and live yogurt help to rebalance the gut bacteria; if appropriate address any emotional tension.

Pain

Pain in the digestive tract can range from an occasional dull ache to intermittent or constant sharp pain. The type of pain indicates the type of problem. Any extreme and acute pain requires immediate professional attention although any form of recurring digestive pain should be investigated.

Most commonly digestive pain is caused by flatulence

Chamomile	
Cramp Bark	
Fennel	in equal parts

Any other carminative and anti-spasmodic herbs should resolve isolated instances.

In the following, specific digestive complaints are reviewed sequentially from the mouth to the anus.

Stomatitis

This very common condition is characterized by:
- an inflamed and sore mouth, with or without mouth ulcers
- the mucous membrane of the mouth is red and swollen

■ profuse salivation accompanied by bad breath

■ possibly a slight fever.

The condition is generally associated with being 'run down'. It often occurs with other digestive disorders and after respiratory infections, antibiotic treatment, stress or with menstruation.

Treatment should aim to improve general health while at the same time addressing the specific cause.

To treat a sore mouth or any mouth ulcers a mouth wash (infusion) used frequently and regularly is very effective:

Marigold	1 part
Marshmallow root	1 part
Red Sage	2 parts

If stress is a marked feature, support the nervous system with relaxing nervines or nervine tonics.

Echinacea and plenty of Garlic, fresh fruit and foods rich in zinc and B vitamins strengthen the immune system. Live yogurt may be considered in order to rebalance digestive bacteria. Spicy and acidic foods should be avoided until symptoms have subsided.

Gastritis

Prolonged demands on the stomach in the form of bad eating habits and a diet high in irritants (alcohol, coffee, cigarettes) can lead to acute or chronic inflammation of the stomach lining. Other causes of gastritis are acute infections of, for example, the tonsils or teeth or long-term nervous tension and stress.

Gastritis can be acute or chronic and manifests with:

■ impaired appetite

■ pain in the abdomen

■ nausea

■ possibly vomiting.

Herbally, the irritated membranes need to be soothed and healed. A basic infusion suitable for individual adaptations would be:

Agrimony	1 part
Marshmallow root	2 parts
Meadowsweet	1 part

If there is much flatulence and muscular spasm add a carminative.

If stress is a significant factor, add a suitable nervine.

The dietary aim is to remove all foods and drink that cause irritation of chemical or mechanical origin as well as fatty foods and extremes of temperature.

■ Chemical irritants are:
- acidic foods, such as vinegar, pickles
- alcohol
- coffee
- hot spices
- cigarettes

■ Mechanical irritants are all foods high in fibre.

These should be avoided for a while and only gradually reintroduced when improvement is continous.

Gastric ulcer

Continued irritation will lead to reduced resistance of the stomach lining to the eroding effects of digestive juices, especially pepsin, and the eventual apperance of an ulcer.

Most noticeably there will be:

■ loss of appetite

■ sharp stomach pain that improves with food as it absorbs the gastric juices

■ gradual weight loss.

Suggestions for gastritis should be followed. Long-term changes in diet and lifestyle, including stress reduction are likely to be needed in order to achieve complete healing.

Peptic or duodenal ulcer

The walls of the duodenum will become inflamed and ulcerated if, over a long period of time, the highly acidic stomach contents enter the alkaline environment of the small intestines.

Emotional stress is a significant factor in the development of peptic ulcers as the valve between the stomach and the duodenum is subject to emotional tension via the autonomic nervous system.

As with gastric ulcers, there is:

- loss of appetite
- gradual weight loss
- gnawing pain that is relieved with foods
- painful attacks at night are characteristic
- often there is also general loss of vitality and increasing debility.

The suggestions for herbal healing and diet are similar to those given for gastric ulcers. In addition, it needs to be considered that toxins from the ulcer, in the same way as nutrients, are also entering the bloodstream. This needs to be addressed in any herbal mixture by including immunostimulants and lymphatic cleansers such as Echinacea, Marigold and Cleavers. A good basic tea would consist of:

Agrimony	
Lemon Balm	
Marigold	
Marshmallow	
Meadowsweet	in equal parts

In addition to following dietary advice and herbal treatment, the causes of the ulcer, most commonly stress and tension, need to be assessed and effectively addressed. For long-term healing this may well require some significant lifestyle changes.

Gastro-enteritis

This is a non-specific term for a number of infections caused mostly by viruses and bacteria leading to inflammation in any part of the small intestines.

Symptoms of gastro-enteritis are:

■ sudden onset of abdominal pain
■ nausea
■ vomiting and diarrhoea.

Suggestions given for duodenal ulcers should be sufficient in most cases.

Appendicitis

The appendix, a small offshoot of the intestine at the junction of the small intestine and the colon, can become inflamed and infected.

A sudden attack with acute lower right abdominal pain calls for immediate medical attention as a burst appendix can be life threatening.

A chronic infection, often described as a rumbling appendix, can manifest with:

■ episodes of recurring dull pain in the lower right abdomen
■ loss of appetite
■ nausea
■ a rise in temperature and possible vomiting
■ often a history of constipation.

Foremost, dietary changes need to take place to eliminate any sources of infection. A diet high in fruit and vegetables and plenty of fluid to move the bowel contents, plenty of Garlic in case of infection and a little live yoghurt to address imbalances in gut flora are necessary. In addition, an infusion to support the body's healing is important:

Agrimony	1 part
Echinacea or Marigold	2 parts
Chamomile	1 part

Ulcerative colitis

This is a non-specific inflammatory disease of the mucus membranes of the colon. The lining undergoes steady erosion with ulcer formation.

The usual manifestations are:

■ increased frequency in bowel movements
■ spells of bloody diarrhoea
■ abdominal cramping
■ cracks or ulcers at the corner of the mouth
■ attacks may be acute.

A combination of soothing and healing herbs with an astringent component will be needed as will be support for the nervous system.

Choose from demulcents such as Comfrey and Marshmallow, healing and astringent herbs such as Marigold and Agrimony and nervines such as Lemon Balm, Skullcap and Lavender. Depending on the circumstances it may also be necessary to include anti-microbials such as Echinacea and Garlic.

In the acute condition a useful mixture drunk 4–5 times a day is:

Agrimony	
Echinacea	
Lemon Balm	
Marigold	
Marshmallow root	in equal parts

For long-term maintenance a tasty and effective mixture is:

Lemon Balm	
Marigold	
Peppermint	in equal parts

The main food item that causes an allegic reaction in this situation is cow's milk and all its products. It needs to be strictly avoided. Goat and soya milk are usually acceptable substitutes. As in gastric ulcers (see above), the diet should be devoid of chemical and mechanical irritants, fats and extremes of temperature. Meals should be small and taken frequently to reduce any undue burden on the digestive system.

Irritable bowel syndrome

IBS is characterized by disordered bowel movements.

Common indicators include:

- bowel movements vary between constipation and diarrhoea or painless urgent diarrhoea
- mucus may be passed between movements
- variable degrees of abdominal pain over areas of the colon, ranging from intermittent colicky pain to a continuous dull ache
- associated symptoms: nausea, bloating, headaches, anxiety and depression
- symptoms tend to be worse in the morning or during/after eating
- problems at night are unusual.

Treatment aims at protecting the mucous membrane with demulcent and anti-inflammatory herbs regulating gastric secretions with astringents and improving peristalsis with anti-spasmodics. Support for the nervous system is also needed.

The following is a pleasant mixture which may be taken long term:

Agrimony	1 part
Chamomile	1 part
Cinnamon	1 part
Lemon Balm	1 part
Peppermint	2 parts

Some people find Dandelion coffee (roasted Dandelion root) effective for alleviation of symptoms. The regular use of Linseed

(1–2 teaspoons per day) helps to balance bowel action by acting as a demulcent bulk laxative that also absorbs increased gastric secretions.

Irritating foods such as bran, coffee, alcohol and dairy produce, especially cheese, should be avoided.

The liver

The liver plays an integral part in maintaining our health. Most disorders or diseases in any part of the body are likely also to affect the liver and be reflected in the efficiency of its multifaceted functioning. Equally, liver dysfunction is likely to manifest itself elsewhere in the body; for instance pre-menstrual complaints can be the result of either a hormonal imbalance or the reduced ability of the liver to inactivate hormones.

The liver can be supported by the use of hepatics, which are bitter herbs that especially act on it.

A general detoxifying mixture consists of:

Burdock root	1 part
Dandelion root	2 parts
Nettle	1 part

Drunk over a period of time, it is effective in improving liver and eliminative functions in general.

Much use was made in the past of 'spring tonics' based on early spring herbs to help in the detoxification of the body and the general strengthening of the liver.

A very pleasant mixture is:

Cleavers	
Dandelion leaf	
Nettle	in equal parts

The herbs can also be used in salads, soups or juices.

This should be complemented by a diet that decreases any digestive burden on the liver. Avoid alcohol, coffee, fat and fatty foods, such as fried or roasted foods and cheese. Instead eat plenty of fresh fruit and vegetables and drink plenty of water. Carrots, beetroot and apples are liver foods and can easily be prepared as fresh juice.

10 | THE URINARY SYSTEM

The urinary system is predominantly concerned with the maintenance of a constant, healthy internal environment – homeostasis – in the body.

In western societies the lifestyle and diet are frequently not in harmony with either our inner or outer environments. Hence, the role of the kidneys assumes a particularly important place in the maintenance of our well-being and the prevention of ill-health.

Within a holistic approach, herbs for the urinary system are not relevant only for problems within the system, but may also be significant in supporting the body's cleansing mechanisms through the bowels, skin and lungs as well as the kidneys.

Anatomy and physiology

The urinary system consists of:
- two kidneys
- two ureters
- bladder
- urethra.

The most important function of the urinary system is to regulate the body's water balance by producing and excreting urine and reabsorbing vital fluids. It also regulates the body's chemical composition and its acid/alkaline balance.

Kidneys

The function of the kidneys is to separate certain waste products such as urea from protein metabolism and salt and uric acid from the blood. This helps to maintain the blood at a constant level of

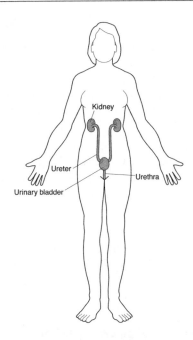

chemical composition despite the great variation in diet and fluid intake. As blood circulates in the kidneys, a large quantity of water, salts, urea and glucose are filtered and all glucose, most of the water and salt and some urea are reabsorbed from here into the bloodstream for our bodily requirements.

It is estimated that 150–180 litres of fluid are filtered daily by the kidneys but only about 1.5 litres of this leaves the body as urine. It is due to the kidneys' ability to differentiate between waste products and valuable substances that a healthy urinary system holds such an important place in our well-being. In addition, the kidneys are involved in the production of renin, a hormone that can cause constriction of the body's arteries leading to an increase in blood pressure. Hence, a persistent kidney weakness may account for high blood pressure.

Ureters

The ureters are muscular tubes which pass the urine from the kidneys to the bladders.

Bladder

Substances that our body doesn't need are eliminated as urine. Muscles, which we learn to control in early childhood, keep the bladder firmly closed while it gradually extends as it fills. The full bladder sends a message to the brain telling it of the need to urinate. We pass urine from the bladder through the urethra.

To help flush out the urinary system and prevent the concentration of unwanted substances in the urine, it is important to drink plenty of water, approximately two litres per day. A persistently concentrated urine can lead to irritation, infection and formation of gravel and stones in kidneys and bladder.

Urethra

The urethra passes from the bladder to the outside; it is approximately 7 cm long in women and 20 cm in men. This anatomical difference accounts for the frequency of cystitis in women and urethritis in men.

Herbs for the urinary system

Diuretics

Diuretics are herbs that increase the secretion, flow and elimination of urine. Most herbs for the urinary system are diuretic in addition to other actions. The most useful diuretic is Dandelion leaf but also consider others such as:

Borage	Horsetail	Ribwort
Cleavers	Marigold	Yarrow
Elderflower	Nettle	

Antiseptics

These are needed in any situation where an infection in the urinary system is present:

Bearberry	Hydrangea	Ribwort
Echinacea	Marigold	Thyme
Garlic	Meadowsweet	Yarrow

Demulcents

Demulcents soothe urinary membranes when they are irritated and inflamed:

Comfrey	Marshmallow
Hydrangea	Ribwort
Liquorice	

Astringents

These will arrest bleeding in any part of the urinary system and help heal damaged membranes. (N.B. All bleeding from the urinary system needs the diagnosis and attention of a medical practitioner.)

Horsetail
Ladies' Mantle
Ribwort

Complaints of the urinary system

The urinary system is prone to conditions associated with infections, irritation and inflammation of the membrane lining of tissues such as the bladder. Reduced kidney function can manifest in the formation of mineral deposits or high blood pressure, but is beyond our scope here.

Urinary tract infection

Due to the anatomical differences in the urethra between female and male (see Anatomy and Physiology), women are more frequently affected by urinary tract infections. Infections can be caused by bowel bacteria entering the tract as well as vaginal infections such as thrush and chlamydia spreading to the urethra and bladder.

Cystitis

Inflammation and infection of the bladder is characterized by:

■ burning or stinging pain on passing urine;
■ the need to urinate frequently, and often urgently, although not much water may be passed;

- the urine may be strong smelling, cloudy or at times pink, which indicates the presence of blood and requires medical attention.

Symptoms of cystitis can occur even if there is no infection confirmed by urine analysis. If you are prone to recurrent bouts of cystitis, consider the following:

- Chemical irritants, soap, bubble bath, chlorine in swimming pools etc. can lead to irritation of the urethra.
- Certain contraceptives such as the diaphragm, spermicidal creams and condoms can irritate the urethra and increase pressure on the bladder.
- Hormonal changes during the menstrual cycle, pregnancy and menopause can relax the muscle of the bladder making it more susceptible to infections.

Thrush is often implicated in causing cystitis in women. Recurrent cystitis may also indicate diabetes and other long-term health problems.

The key to treating cystitis is to dilute the irritating effects of the urine with plenty of fluid, about 2–3 litres per day, in the form of water or herbal teas.

Acute cystitis

Marshmallow
Thyme or Bearberry
Yarrow   in equal parts

Five or 6 cups of this infusion can be drunk throughout the day.

Cranberry juice can be very effective in readjusting the body's acid/alkaline balance and may resolve the problem if an attack was preceded by a time of poor diet and lifestyle.

Once the acute symptoms recede, the mixture can be changed and drunk regularly until all symptoms have cleared up.

Marigold	
Ribwort	
Yarrow	in equal parts

Avoid the following food items during an attack as they irritate the delicate membranes of the urinary system:

- tea
- coffee
- alcohol
- sugar
- spicy foods

Urethritis and Prostatitis

Urethritis, the inflammation of the urethra, and prostatitis, an infection of the prostate gland, benefit from the same approach as cystitis.

Pyelonephritis

Infections from the bladder and urethra can spread to cause an infection of the kidneys. Kidney infections are a serious problem and medical help should be sought immediately.

Characteristic symptoms are:

- fever
- lower back pain that can be intense and incapacitating
- headache
- general malaise.

The herbal approach combines strategies discussed for cystitis with general treatment for fever and infections.

Water retention

Accumulation of fluid beneath the skin indicates that the kidneys do not excrete enough fluid from the body. The excess water often collects around the ankles, fingers, breasts and the abdomen.

Water retention can be a complication of urinary and circulatory diseases or diabetes and frequently occurs pre-menstrually. To treat the fluid retention effectively, the underlying causes need to be established and addressed.

For simple water retention, such as pre-menstrually, a salt-free diet and the use of Nettle, Yarrow or Dandelion herb tea for a few days is likely to resolve the problem.

11 | THE MUSCULOSKELETAL SYSTEM

Our skeleton constitutes the framework of our body. It is largely covered by muscles attached to bones, thus enabling us to move. The health of this system depends on the structure and the use we make of it, as well as our emotional and physical well-being, diet and lifestyle – that is, the health of our body as a whole.

Anatomy and physiology

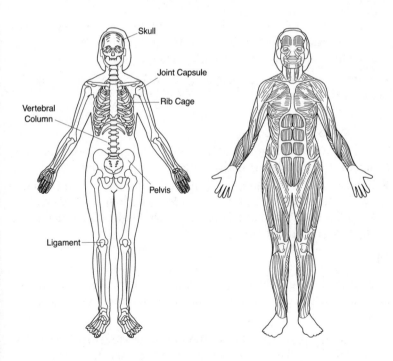

The musculoskeletal system consists of:

■ skeleton; bone; muscle.

Skeleton

The skeleton has two main functions:

■ It protects a range of organs e.g. the skull protects the brain, the spinal column protects the spinal cord, the ribcage protects the heart and lungs.

■ Through the arrangement of bones, joints, tendons and muscles, it allows for our movements.

The skeleton comprises approximately 206 bones.

Bone

Bone is a dry dense tissue made up of 25% water, 30% organic material and 45% mineral, mostly calcium phosphate and some magnesium salt.

In addition to providing protection and movement, bones also provide for attachment of muscles and the production of red and some white blood cells in the bone marrow.

A **joint** is a junction of two or more bones. Depending on the mobility, joints are divided into three groups:

■ Fixed joints, such as sutures between the skull bones, have almost no movement.

■ Slightly moveable joints held together by strong ligaments, but separated by pads consisting of cartilage e.g. pubic bones.

■ Freely moveable joints e.g. hip joint, elbow, knee and ankles, are covered by a fibrous capsule, which is linked with a synovial membrane and filled with synovial fluid. The joint is supported by ligament.

Muscle

The function of muscle is to permit movement, hence most muscles are attached to bone. There are about 640 named muscles in the body.

Each muscle consists of elastic fibres collected together in bundles, often bound together but always enclosed in a sheath. This extends at either end to form a strong tendon which attaches the muscle to the bone.

There are two types of muscle:

■ Voluntary muscles, such as those used for walking, sitting, chewing, are under conscious control.

■ Involuntary muscles, involved in heart function, breathing and digestion, are not under conscious control.

Muscle action results from a stimulus received from a motor nerve. This nerve stimulus causes chemical changes such as breakdown of fats, glucose and glycogen, which in turn provides the energy required for its action. The waste products created by this process, mostly urea and lactic acid, are eliminated through the veins and the lymphatic system.

Muscular activity not only generates the energy needed for its function but also heat which warms the body. Through the involuntary action of shivering more heat is produced by the muscle should it be necessary to counteract falling body temperature.

Herbs for the musculoskeletal system

Alteratives

These herbs favourably change blood and lymph to detoxify and renew body tissue. Most arthritic and rheumatic conditions benefit from the cleansing action of these herbs:

Celery seed	Marigold
Cleavers	Nettle

Anti-inflammatories

These help to reduce inflammation and enable the body to heal and regenerate affected tissues. They are particularly relevant in arthritic and rheumatic conditions.

Comfrey	Meadowsweet
Liquorice	White Willow

Anti-rheumatics

These help to relieve the discomfort of rheumatism and arthritis. Many of the herbs listed here have other primary indications and choice should be based on the holistic assessment of individual needs:

Burdock   Meadowsweet
Celery seed   Nettle
Dandelion   Yarrow
Lavender

Diuretics

Diuretics help the kidneys in the elimination of metabolic waste and toxins. In chronic inflammatory conditions a diuretic should be included to ensure effective excretion of the by-products of inflammation and metabolism:

Celery seed   Nettle
Dandelion leaf   Yarrow

Digestive bitters

These ensure the effective function of the digestive system including elimination through the bowels:

Burdock root
Celery seed
Dandelion root

Circulatory stimulants

These herbs improve the peripheral circulation and increase the blood flow to the muscles and joints. This in turn leads to more efficient removal of toxins and relieves inflammation and congestion:

Ginger
Rosemary
Yarrow

Nervines

Chronic musculoskeletal problems are often accompanied by chronic pain. While anti-inflammatory herbs relieve some of the pain, nervines with their analgesic action may also be helpful:

Chamomile   St John's Wort
Skullcap   Wood Betony

Complaints of the musculoskeletal system

Conditions in this system tend to be caused by either structural problems or by a mostly long-term and gradual decline of general physical and emotional well-being. It is the latter that is our concern here.

To approach conditions manifesting in the bones, joints and muscles holistically, digestive function and all the pathways of elimination such as skin, kidneys, lymphatics, and lungs have to be addressed, as does the circulation. Over time herbs together with an appropriate diet are likely to help heal and rebalance disturbances contributing to problems in this area.

Rheumatism and arthritis

As there are numerous different types of arthritis and rheumatism, we focus on the commonalities in causes, herbal treatment and dietary changes.

Common symptoms in affected joints are:

- tenderness and pain
- stiffness
- swelling and redness
- systemic inflammation with increased temperature and general malaise.

One of the causes of these conditions is a long-term accumulation of toxins and waste products in the affected areas. Generally, processed foods full of preservatives and additives and foods that cause allergic reactions, particularly gluten in wheat, barley, rye and oats and cow's milk dairy produce are well known to cause and aggravate arthritic and rheumatic complaints.

It is most important to recognize that these conditions result from the body's inability to deal with the burdens caused by a number of different stresses, both emotional and physical, ranging from wrong diet and lifestyle to long-term emotional pressures.

In general terms, food should be organic and as fresh as possible. Foods that cause acidic reactions in the body should be avoided, such as meats, eggs, vinegar, and pickles as should acidic foods such as tomatoes, rhubarb, currants and gooseberries. People with rheumatoid arthritis often have sensitivities to citrus fruits, oranges, lemon and grapefruit, especially in the form of juice, while sufferers of osteo-arthritis tend to have sensitivities to foods from the Nightshade family such as tomatoes, aubergine, red and green peppers and potatoes. Refined carbohydrates, sugars, coffee, tea, alcohol and salt also contribute to toxic overloads and should be avoided; instead fruit and vegetables should be eaten in plenty. Fish, white meat, pulses, wholegrain rice and root vegetables are likewise recommended. Plenty of fluids should be drunk daily to help flush out the system.

Holistic herbal treatment aims to improve a person's overall well-being and vitality to enable the body to deal with the range of symptoms commonly encountered and to initiate the long term and gradual process of cleansing the body and reversing some of the degenerative development.

The following basic mixture should be adjusted to suit the individual needs:

Celery seed
Willow Bark
Yarrow   in equal parts
If there is sluggish elimination of toxins through the bowel, choose from bitter anti-rheumatics or digestive bitters such as Dandelion root or Burdock root. Add alteratives for the lymphatic system and consider Hawthorn and Ginger should the circulation need support. If required add a suitable nervine.

In addition, external remedies can be used locally to ease stiffness, pain and inflammation. A warming oil can be prepared with Ginger and Cayenne or Peppermint or Winter Green oil can be used to make a cooling preparation. Infused oils of Comfrey or St John's Wort are effective in alleviating muscle and nerve pains.

When creating a suitable environment for physical healing to take place it is equally important to address a person's emotional well-being. Letting go of emotional negativity and rigid emotional patterns can contribute to the healing process as much as cleansing herbs. Relaxation exercises, meditation, yoga and other techniques are also vital to support the easing of emotional and physical stresses that have a long-term contribution to the development of the condition.

Gout

Gout is an inflammatory reaction to micro-crystals of sodium urate building up in the body.

Acute episodes:

■ start suddenly and at night
■ after injury, surgery, excessive food or alcohol intake
■ are usually confined to one joint, especially the big toe.

The use of anti-rheumatics and diuretics will help to support elimination especially through the kidneys. Celery seed is particularly effective.

A low-acid diet is recommended. Some fish such as sardines, anchovies, shellfish and crab, as well as liver, kidney and beans should be avoided as they are high in purines that the body metabolizes to uric acid. Coffee, tea, and alcohol should be replaced with plenty of water and cleansing herb teas.

Bursitis

Bursitis is the chronic or acute inflammation of a bursa. The bursa are sac-like cavities filled with fluid between larger tendons and bones. They facilitate movement of joints and minimize friction between the different parts.

The causes of bursitis are unknown, although it may be caused by overuse, trauma and infections.

Commonly affected joints are in the shoulder, knees and elbows.

Herbs to ease the inflammation and pain are helpful as are local applications suggested under arthritis.

Sprains

Sprains of ligaments and tendons due to accidents can be exceedingly painful. Hot applications with stimulating herbs or added to hot baths, e.g. Ginger compresses, increase the local circulation and facilitate repair. Comfrey, as an ointment or poultice, helps to reduce swelling, bruises and pain and facilitates the healing of damaged tissues, such as muscle, tendon or ligament.

12 | THE REPRODUCTIVE SYSTEM

For the female or male reproductive system to be functioning smoothly our physical, emotional and mental well-being must be balanced. If our sense of self, self-esteem and identity as individuals are well integrated into our lives we are more likely to be thriving as a whole person and hence tend to suffer less from reproductive health problems.

A balanced diet also has major repercussions especially on women's health as much of our physical and emotional well-being can be subject to hormonal imbalances and fluctuations; these in turn are exacerbated by nutritional deficiencies.

Due to the differing complexities in anatomy, physiology and function between the female and male reproduction system, a certain imbalance in detail in the following discussion of the systems is inevitable.

THE MALE REPRODUCTIVE SYSTEM

Anatomy and physiology

The main organs are:

■ testes
■ scrotums
■ penis.

Testes

The testes or testicles, are the most significant male reproductive glands. They have two principal functions:

■ the development of the sperm
■ the secretion of the testosterone, the male sex hormone.

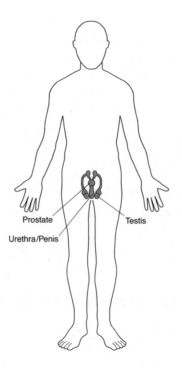

Prostate

Testis

Urethra/Penis

Scrotum

The scrotum, a sac-like organ in which the testes are contained, allows for the development of sperm to take place in an environment that has a slightly lower temperature than the body.

Penis

The penis, a gland which consists of erectile tissues, is suspended in front of the scrotum.

The penis and scrotum constitute the external genital organs; a number of glands and a series of ducts form part of the internal structures.

The male reproductive system has four aspects:

■ the secretion of male sex hormones
■ the sexual response
■ the formation and maintenance of sperm
■ transport of the sperm cells to the female reproductive organs.

Herbs for the male reproductive system

Antiseptics

Antiseptics may be needed in any situation where there is an infection in the system:

Bearberry	Ribwort
Hydrangea	Thyme
Marigold	Yarrow

Demulcents

These soothe mucous membranes and may be indicated in irritation and inflammation:

Comfrey
Marshmallow
Ribwort

Diuretics

These herbs help to detoxify the system by increasing the secretion and elimination of urine:

Bearberry	Nettle
Horsetail	Ribwort
Hydrangea	Yarrow

Astringents

Astringents will help to heal damaged membranes:

Horsetail
Nettle
Ribwort

Tonics

These are called for to strengthen tissues and organs and to balance overall functions.

Hydrangea
Nettle

Complaints of the male reproductive system

The main problems associated with this system originate in the prostate gland. Infections or enlargements are the most common complaints.

Prostatitis

Acute prostatitis, a bacterial infection of the prostate gland, is characterized by:

■ fever
■ urinary frequency and urgency, especially at night
■ low back pain
■ burning on urination
■ general malaise.

Treatment is as for acute cystitis (see Urinary system) and should be started promptly to avoid the development of chronic prostatitis.

In chronic prostatitis the symptoms are variable. Most commonly experienced are:

■ low back pain
■ urinary frequency and urgency
■ pain or irritation.

Relapsing urinary tract infections such as cystitis are particularly common.

The following mixture drunk regularly 2–3 times a day over several weeks should help to clear the problem:

Nettle
Ribwort
Thyme
Yarrow   in equal parts

Benign enlargement of the prostate

This condition leads to obstruction of the urethra and interference with the flow of urine. It commonly affects men over 50 and is thought to be due to alteration in the hormonal balance associated with ageing.

Common symptoms include:

■ progressive urinary frequency and urgency
■ nocturia (the need to pass water during the night)
■ decreased size and force of urinary stream leading to hestitancy
■ sensations of incomplete emptying of bladder
■ dribbling and incontinence.

Hydrangea is a herb of choice for this situation:

Horsetail	1 part
Hydrangea	2 parts
Nettle	1 part

An infusion can be drunk 2–3 times a day over a period to help restore effective function.

Zinc has shown to reduce the size of the prostate gland and zinc-rich foods such as pumpkin and sunflower seeds, whole grains including rice, dried fruit, dairy products, beans and onion and garlic should be actively incorporated into the diet.

In addition, soya is said to have prostate-protective effects. To increase soya in the diet also helps the body to utilize zinc as a high protein intake is required to do so.

THE FEMALE REPRODUCTIVE SYSTEM

Anatomy and physiology

A woman's body is superbly developed and adaptable to fulfilling various functions at different times of a woman's life.

The main female reproductive organs are:

- the ovaries
- the Fallopian tubes
- the uterus, including the cervix
- the vagina, vulva and clitoris
- the breasts.

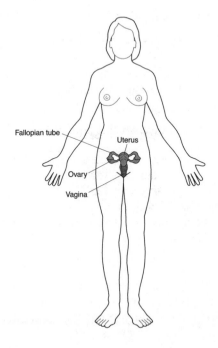

Fallopian tube
Uterus
Ovary
Vagina

The ovaries

The ovaries, the primary internal organs, are each about the size of an almond and consist of a great number of small sacs called the ovarian follicles. Each follicle contains an egg.

The ovaries have two main functions:

■ to develop the eggs and release one approximately every 28 days throughout a woman's reproductive life

■ to produce the hormones oestrogen and progesterone which influence secondary female characteristics and control uterine changes during the menstrual cycle.

The Fallopian tubes

The Fallopian tubes transport the egg from the ovaries to the womb.

The uterus

The uterus is a pear-shaped organ in the centre of the pelvis in between the bladder to the front and the rectum to the back. The lower part of the uterus, the cervix, fits into the upper part of the vagina. The wall of the uterus is about 2.5cm thick and consists mostly of mucous membrane called endometrium, which is extremely sensitive to oestrogen and progesterone. The uterus serves as a site for the growth and nourishment of a baby during pregnancy.

The vagina, vulva and clitoris

The vagina is an elastic, muscular membrane. It transmits male sperm to the uterus and acts as a birth canal for the newborn. The external genitals, collectively called vulva, comprise the labia and clitoris; they are located within the perineum. Both the vagina and the vulva are richly supplied with muscles, nerves and blood vessels.

The breasts

The breasts consist of fatty, fibrous tissue and associated nerves, blood and lymphatic vessels.

At puberty, the increased secretion of oestrogen influences the enlargement of the nipple and areola and increases fat tissue in the breast resulting in variable breast sizes.

The lymphatic vessels are an important part of the breasts as they drain fat from the milk produced during breast feeding and transport infected material or cancerous cells from the breast to other parts of the body.

The female reproductive system has six different aspects:

- the secretion of sex hormones
- the sexual response
- production and transportation of eggs
- receipt and transport of male sperm to the uterus
- preparation of the uterus for and maintenance of the developing baby during pregnancy
- initial feeding of the newborn during lactation.

The menstrual cycle

A woman's reproductive cycle begins at about the age of 12 and ends at about 45–55 years of age. Each cycle lasts approximately 28 days, although a cycle as short as 21 days and as long as 40–45 days is not uncommon and in itself no cause for concern.

The cycle is initiated and maintained by hormones and characterized by the breakdown of the lining of the uterus (endometrium) and subsequent menstrual blood loss. Throughout the cycle significant changes in follicular and endometrial structure take place that serve to develop and release a female germ cell for possible fertilization and to prepare the uterus for implantation of a fertilized egg.

The menstrual period, consisting of the first 5–7 days of the cycle, is characterized by blood loss due to the disintegration of endometrial tissue. On about the fifth day of the menstrual cycle, influenced by hormones from the ovarian follicle, the endometrium begins to regrow.

Herbs for the female reproductive system

A multitude of herbs are found to benefit the female reproductive system throughout the different stages of a woman's life.

Uterine tonics

These are healers in the true sense. They hold a special place among the herbs for women as they aid the whole woman by toning, strengthening and regulating reproductive functions, associated hormones and the well-being of the womb and ovaries. Choose from the following brief list of my favourites, but bear in mind that, as always, each herb is unique in its range of influence and action:

Ladies' Mantle	Sage
Marigold	Yarrow
Raspberry	

Emmenagogues

These herbs initiate and promote menstrual flow through the stimulation and elimination of congested endometrium. They may be indicated in pelvic congestion manifesting in period pains. Due to their stimulating and, at times, irritating action, emmenagogues are contra-indicated in pregnancy (for complete list, see Chapter 19). In addition to the listed uterine tonics, the following herbs are also powerful emmenagogues:

Cinnamon
Ginger
Rosemary

Hormonal regulators

These adjust the balance of female sex hormones by either stimulating or initiating the release of hormones, especially oestrogen and progesterone, from the pituitary gland or the ovaries. Hence, they are often called for in menstrual and gynaecological conditions that are associated with hormonal imbalances:

Chaste Tree	Sage
Ladies' Mantle	Yarrow

In addition Watercress and Alfalfa help to regulate pituitary function as do Evening Primrose oil and Borage seed oil (also called Starflower oil). (See also Uterine tonics).

Astringents

These are often used in the context of heavy menstrual bleeding.

Ladies' Mantle	Sage
Raspberry	Yarrow
Nettle	

Demulcents

Demulcents help to heal and soothe irritated and inflamed mucous membranes.

Marigold
Marshmallow
Ribwort

Antiseptics and anti-microbials

These may be called for in inflammations and infections in any part of the reproductive system.

Cinnamon	Sage
Marigold	Yarrow
Ribwort	

General antiseptics and anti-microbials or urinary antiseptics are also usually appropriate.

Alteratives

Due to their ability to detoxify the lymphatic system and promote the renewal of the body tissue, alteratives are often used when holistically addressing gynaecological conditions. For general suggestions see the chapter on the lymph system. Alternatives with an affinity for the reproductive system are:

Marigold
Nettle
Red Clover

Nervines

Supporting the functions of the nervous system, nervines often facilitate and ease the functions of the reproductive system in its many manifestations. Relaxing anti-spasmodic herbs are particularly effective in any condition associated with muscular cramp and spasm, and nervine tonics should be considered in conditions related to long-term tension manifesting in the reproductive system:

Cramp Bark	Rosemary
Lavender	Skullcap
Lemon Balm	Wood Betony

Complaints of the female reproductive system

Nature's rhythms manifest themselves in the changing seasons, the ebb and flow of the tides and the phases of the moon. Likewise, our own rhythms are characterized by cyclical and spiral patterns – from the ebb and flow of our monthly hormones to the spiral of hormonal changes throughout much of our lives.

A multitude of influences and events ranging from the individual and personal to external, such as social and environmental, will have a profound impact on our hormonal patterns and fluctuations. Our overall well-being depends on recognizing this as much as on the ability to take control of our bodies and our lives in the face of continuing obstacles.

Here, I look briefly at common problems associated with the menstrual cycle during different times of a woman's life, breast problems and infections.

To discuss issues relevant to pregnancy, childbirth and breast feeding are beyond the scope of this book.

Menstrual health

A great deal of information can be gained about a woman's health by assessing the following:

■ *The cycle*

Much is said and written about the normal length of the cycle. Although a 28-day cycle is assumed to be normal, healthy and correct, the experiences of most women do not confirm this. Instead, cycles commonly range from 21 days to about 40–45 days, give or take 1–2 days' variation between each cycle. On charting our cycle, many so-called irregular cycles reveal their own rhythm and regularity hidden under layers of unhelpful assumptions.

The menstrual cycle, however, can be disturbed by many factors, with hormonal or emotional imbalances being the most common. Amenorrhoea, the lack of menstruation, for more than three to four months should be investigated.

■ *Colour of the blood*

In health, menstrual blood should be bright red and vibrant in colour. It indicates ease of circulation and good blood supply to the uterus, ovaries and the pelvic area in general.

Lightly coloured pinkish blood throughout your period may indicate poor general circulation with low blood pressure and possibly anaemia. Dark red or brownish blood throughout your period is likely to imply poor pelvic circulation, often together with sluggish bowels and a fair degree of menstrual pain either before the onset of bleeding or on the first day of the period.

If your diet contains a high percentage of refined carbohydrates, meats, alcohol and chemical additives, the colour of your blood is likely to be darker. This also tends to be the case during illness or while convalescing. Hence a well-balanced diet high in fruit and vegetables, if not vegetarian, contributes to healthy menstrual blood as well as overall health.

■ *Consistency of blood*

Menstrual blood clots can be variable ranging from the size of a small coin to that of the palm of the hand. Most smallish clots are likely to go unnoticed although discharging a number of large clots can be distressing and painful. Like the colour of the blood, clots too are indicators of pelvic blood flow – the more clots and the larger their size, the more congested the pelvic area tends to be. Other symptoms such as headaches, constipation and fluid retention are often additional indicators.

■ *Flow and loss of blood*

The average period lasts about 5–7 days with the heaviest flow a few hours after onset and on the second day, trailing off at the end of days 4 and 5.

Should you have to change your pad or tampon routinely more than every 2–3 hours during the day and more than once at night for more than 1–2 days your blood flow is likely to be heavy. If you need to change only once or twice a day your blood flow is slight. Check for other indicators of low blood pressure and anaemia.

As you get used to reading and interpreting this information in a holistic way, it will provide you with valuable indications of your general well-being.

Disturbances of the menstrual cycle

Irregular periods

A woman is said to have an irregular cycle when her periods fluctuate with no distinct pattern, length of bleeding is variable and the amount of blood lost changes with each menstruation.

Irregular cycles tend to be related to hormonal imbalances with additional factors contributing.

The most common causes are:

■ low thyroid function
■ antibiotics and other drugs
■ dietary deficiencies
■ weight fluctuations
■ long-term illness
■ prolonged stress and trauma
■ lifestyle changes such as moving home or travel.

For best results, a holistic assessment is needed in order to harmonise an irregular cycle. Here are some general ideas.

■ If you feel prolonged stress is your main underlying problem, refer to the section on stress.
■ If you feel you suffer from chronic illness, assess your needs in this context; evaluate any medication together with your practitioner.

■ Ask to be tested for thyroid function or dietary deficiencies, if you suspect either of these to be the cause of the problem.

The following infusion taken over a period of 4–6 months may be helpful to rebalance your cycle.

> Ladies' Mantle
> Marigold
> Yarrow   in equal parts
>
> You may also want to consider additionally taking 15 drops of Chaste Tree tincture in the morning.

Puberty

For adolescent girls, irregular cycles are a common and often disconcerting feature. Over time the cycle should adjust itself as the liver gradually gets used to the additional task of breaking down the hormones thus reducing the intense fluctuations. However, should the irregularity persist, a gentle and pleasantly light tea to help regulate the hormones and support the liver might be helpful:

> Marigold   1 part
> Raspberry leaf   2 parts
>
> Drink twice a day for at least three months.

Menopause

From the age of 45 onwards, changes in the cycle are often initial signs that the menopause is approaching. Between the ages of 45–55 a woman's body is adjusting to declining hormone levels and the take-over process of oestrogen production by the adrenal glands. This leads to a variety of associated symptoms including:

■ very frequent periods or longer times between them

■ heavy bleeding or a lighter and shorter flow

■ hot flushes and night sweats

■ headaches

■ palpitations
■ insomnia
■ mood changes
■ vaginal discharge, irritation or dryness
■ low libido.

Hormone-balancing herbs and herbs with an oestrogen-like action are likely to be the most important, together with herbs to support the adrenal glands, the liver and the nervous system. Don't wait until any menopausal symptoms are severe as it is easier to influence hormones at an early stage.

Ten to 15 drops of Chaste Tree tincture taken in some water on waking may be sufficient to help in the transition especially if you are otherwise healthy and active. At other times, taking Chaste Tree and drinking the following harmonizing tea daily over several months helps in the needed adjustment.

Borage
Marigold
Melissa
Sage
Vervain   in equal parts

If you suffer especially from hot flushes and night sweats, add Hawthorn or Yarrow to balance the circulation.

Painful periods

Period pains can range from a mild dragging sensation in the lower abdomen to severe cramps with vomiting and diarrhoea and other associated symptoms that even strong pain killers may not effectively relieve.

Two types of pain are generally recognized:
■ Spasmodic pains are characterized by:
　– sharp intense cramping pain in the lower abdomen, back and thighs
　– pain usually begins with the period and lasts for 2–3 days

– nausea, vomiting and diarrhoea may be accompanying symptoms

– usually the flow is heavy and the blood bright red.

These pains tend to be caused by strong and frequent uterine contractions while the lining is being shed. The resulting muscular tension in the pelvis reduces the oxygen supply to the uterus, which in turn causes more spasms.

■ Congestive pains are characterized by:

– onset 1–3 days before menstruation

– dull character with a heavy dragging sensation in the pelvis and thighs

– the blood flow is generally heavy, with a dark red colour and variable clotting.

These pains are caused by poor circulation, especially in the pelvic area, with resulting engorged uterine blood vessels.

Both types of pain are commonly improved by stimulating the circulation, balancing hormones and supporting the liver.

A comforting base mixture consists of:

Ladies' Mantle
Marigold
Yarrow or Rosemary   in equal parts
with some Ginger or Cinnamon

This tea is best taken 2–3 times a day for several months, and can be adapted to suit your particular needs.

If you are generally tense and have spasmodic pains, add relaxing herbs such as Lavender, Chamomile or Lemon Balm. If you suspect hormonal imbalance is a significant cause, you may benefit from taking Chaste Tree berries for five to six months. Anti-spasmodic herbs which specifically help to relax spasms and tension in the uterus and cervix can be taken from a few days prior to the onset of the period to relieve body tension. Cramp Bark is especially effective.

Regular but gentle exercise such as walking, swimming or yoga will help to improve pelvic circulation over time and ease menstrual pain. Allow yourself to relax and focus your energies constructively.

Heavy periods

Your periods could be considered heavy if you need to change your pad or tampon every two to three hours during the day, use double protection at night and still need to change or if you bleed considerably for more than two to three days. Should your normal menstrual pattern change and your bleeding become heavier, you should seek advice.

Common causes of heavy bleeding include:

- fibroids
- endometriosis
- low thyroid function
- infections in the reproductive system including intra-uterine devices
- nutritional deficiencies
- menopause.

To control heavy bleeding, your hormones need to be well balanced, uterine arteries need to contract appropriately and the endometrium has to be able to repair itself.

A general mixture to improve heavy bleeding that can be adjusted to suit your particular needs is the following:

Ladies' Mantle
Marigold
Nettle
Yarrow   in equal parts

Drink this tea 2–3 times a day for 4–6 months and use Chaste tree berries in conjunction with it.

If your periods are changing as a result of the menopause, add Sage and Borage. Where stress may be a significant factor support the nervous system with Vervain, Borage or Lemon Balm. If your diet has been particularly poor, cleanse the liver with bitter herbs to aid the hormone metabolism.

Pre-menstrual syndrome (PMS)

PMS refers to a wide range of symptoms which may be present up to 14 days before a period. PMS frequently occurs during puberty, after pregnancy, breast-feeding and after coming off the pill. It is particularly common between the early 30s and early 40s. Many of the symptoms that manifest during this time are the result of hormonal changes after ovulation, especially increasing progesterone or excess oestrogen relative to progesterone.

Physical changes may include:

■ tender swollen breasts
■ water retention with weight gain and swollen hands and feet
■ headaches and migraines
■ painful joints and backache
■ abdominal bloating and digestive upsets
■ poor co-ordination and concentration
■ low energy and sleeping problems
■ hypoglycaemia (low blood sugar levels)
■ increased problems with chronic conditions such as asthma, eczema or candida.

Emotional problems may include:

■ depression
■ irritability, aggression
■ weepiness
■ anxiety, mood swings
■ panic attacks.

To improve your general well-being, make sure your diet is suitable for your needs with plenty of fresh fruit, vegetables, especially watercress and alfalfa, wholegrains, nuts, seeds and pulses. To help readjust your water balance, hormone levels and blood sugar, cut out refined carbohydrates, sugar, salt, tea, coffee, alcohol, cigarettes and chocolates as their consumption contributes to a vicious cycle of hypoglycaemia and adrenal exhaustion. If you are prone to food cravings, hence hypoglycaemia, make sure to eat unrefined carbohydrates at regular, frequent intervals (every two hours) and if needed take a vitamin B complex supplement for a while.

Many women with severe PMS have a diet high in unsaturated animal fats based on dairy produce and meat, which inhibit the formation of prostaglandins. Replace your dairy and meat intake with nuts, seeds and pulses and supplement with Evening Primrose or Borage oil for a while to improve prostaglandin formation.

Address any long-term problems such as food sensitivities as these are likely to exacerbate your pre-menstrual symptoms. Ensure relaxing times for yourself and take regular exercise.

A base herbal preparation for PMS should include herbs to restore hormonal levels especially of oestrogen and progesterone, aid liver function and support the adrenal glands. For mild to moderate PMS, in addition to dietary and lifestyle changes, drink the following mixture 2–3 times a day for 4–6 months:

Borage
Ladies' Mantle
Marigold   in equal parts

In severe and long-standing PMS take 15 drops of the tincture of the Chaste Tree berries in water on waking for four to six months as well.

Breast health

Many women experience breast problems. These may include pre-menstrual tenderness, aching, the occurrence of lumps, cysts and infections. The majority of breast problems are benign, although all problems should, of course, be appropriately investigated.

Regular breast self-examination has proved to be the most effective way of discovering any changes.

Breast cysts

Breast cysts (also called fibrocystic breast disease, fibro-adenosis, cyclical mastalgia, chronic cystic mastitis or benign mammary dysplasia) are fluid-filled pockets causing mostly cyclical symptoms of:

- tenderness
- lumpiness in breast tissue
- change of breast size.

Symptoms vary with the menstrual cycle, are usually worse pre-menstrually and may recede after menstruation. Women between the ages of 20 and 45 are particularly affected. As cysts are subject to hormonal fluctuations, they usually resolve after the menopause.

Excessive oestrogen and prolactin aggravate breast cysts as do chemicals found in tea, coffee, chocolate and cola drinks.

Reduce blood hormone levels by avoiding chemical hormones, for example in the pill and in meats, cut out the above stimulants and reduce fatty foods in your diet to ease any burden on the liver. Take Evening Primrose or Borage seed oil and include Linseed oil in your diet to increase fatty acids. Vitamin E supplements are also often effective. Eat plenty of watercress and alfalfa to help balance pituitary function.

The following herbal mixture drunk regularly for three to four cycles should aid in resolving any residual problems.

Dandelion Root
Ladies' Mantle
Marigold
Nettle
Yarrow   in equal parts

Complement with Chaste Tree berries, if your problems are severe:

Vaginal and vulval infections

Vaginal and vulval infections, collectively called vaginitis, are perhaps among the most common problems experienced by women. The organisms causing vaginitis are normally part of a healthy vaginal environment which has become unbalanced, allowing an infection to take hold. Bacteria, viruses and fungi can all be involved.

Symptoms may include:

■ increased vaginal discharge with a yeasty to fetid smell, runny to thick and heavy texture and white to greenish or brown colour
■ painful, swollen, sore and red vulva
■ itching
■ pain on urination
■ pain on penetrative sexual intercourse.

If you suspect you have an infection, it is best to have a swab taken for accurate analysis. Sexually transmitted diseases such as chlamydia, syphilis and gonorrhoea should be treated in conjunction with orthodox measures. All vaginal and vulval infections need to be addressed promptly as they can lead to serious disease in other parts of the reproductive system.

Lowered resistance is the main cause of any infection, including those in the reproductive system. If you suspect this is the case, address the following:

■ improve your diet and lifestyle
■ consider infections elsewhere in the body
■ treat stress, exhaustion and sleeping problems
■ avoid taking the pill, steroids or antibiotics.

Certain factors affect vaginal and vulval health in particular as they disturb the healthy local environments:

■ Avoid the use of vaginal cosmetics or strong soap in the area.
■ Use mild washing detergents for your underwear and rinse well.
■ Wear only cotton underwear and generally loose clothes as they allow for better circulation.

■ Be meticulous about personal hygiene, although avoid over-
  frequent washing.
■ Encourage your partner also to follow basic hygiene.

The following mixture with cleansing, astringent and anti-
microbial herbs is useful to detoxify and rebalance the reproductive
system. Drink 2–3 cups daily for a period of time:

Cleavers
Echinacea
Ladies' Mantle
Marigold
Thyme   in equal parts

Take garlic frequently to rebalance the vaginal bacteria and
apply natural live yoghurt regularly to ease itching and
soreness.

For a general approach to strengthening the immune system, refer
to the relevant section.

13 | THE NERVOUS SYSTEM

Perhaps it is in the exploration of the nervous system that we can best appreciate the powerful connection and interconnection between the physical, emotional and mental workings of our body as much as our overall well-being. The nervous system is clearly part of our physical entity just as our emotions are reflected in the state of the nervous system. If we suffer from physical ill-health this is likely to impact on our emotional and mental well-being; equally when we are emotionally and mentally unwell, it tends to reflect in our physical health.

Hence, the herbal approach regards the intrinsic relationship between the physical, emotional and mental as well as the spiritual as a vital aspect in the holistic treatment of the whole person.

Anatomy and physiology

The nervous system transmits and receives messages to and from all parts of the body and the brain. It is divided into:

- the central nervous system, which consists of:
  - the brain
  - the spinal cord
- the autonomic nervous system, which consists of:
  - the sympathetic
  - the parasympathetic system.

The functional basis of the nervous system is the nerve cell. This is composed of a nerve cell body with receiving processes called dendrites and its transmitting nerve endings (axon); white nerve fibres are enclosed in a myelin sheath, whereas grey nerve fibres are not.

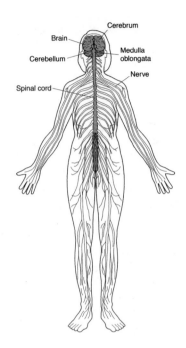

The central nervous system

The brain

The brain, well protected from the outside by the skull, is at the centre of the central nervous system. Inside the skull, the brain is protected by three layered membranes, the meninges.

The brain is composed of three different structures:

■ *The cerebrum*

The cerebrum is arranged in two symmetrical hemispheres. It consists of an outer layer, the cortex, which is the grey brain matter, and the white brain matter made up of nerve fibres, which lies underneath the cortex.

The cerebrum controls voluntary movement and receives and processes conscious sensations. It is the seat of our higher functions such as intelligence and memory and our senses.

■ *The cerebellum*

The cerebellum lies below and behind the cerebrum and is much smaller in size. Like the cerebrum it is also composed of grey and underlying white matter.

The cerebellum is concerned with muscular co-ordination and physical balance.

■ *The medulla oblongata*

The medulla oblongata connects the whole brain with the spinal cord with which it merges; it is made up of interspersed grey and white matter.

The medulla oblongata links the functions of the brain and the spinal cord and is also involved with those parts of the autonomic nervous system that control the heart, respiration, digestive processes etc.

Other parts of the brain include:

■ The *pons varoli* is a bridge of nerve fibres linking all parts of the brain as well as the brain and spinal cord.

■ The *pituitary gland*, situated at the base of the skull, is concerned with our hormonal balance – see endocrine system.

■ The *hypothalamus* exercises an influence over the autonomic nervous system.

The spinal cord

The spinal cord extends four-fifths of the spinal column from the medulla oblongata down through the vertebrae of the spinal column. It is cylindrical in shape with an outer cover made up of cells and blood vessels and an inner centre of nerve fibres.

Nerves

Nerves are bundles of nerve fibres. They conduct all sensations from the body to the brain and spinal cord and conduct motor commands to all the skeletal muscles of the body.

There are 12 pairs of cranial nerves commencing from the base of the brain. A further 31 pairs of spinal nerves branch off throughout the length of the spinal cord. These are often called peripheral nerves. Nerves extending upwards via the spinal column to the brain pass through the medulla oblongata where they cross over – hence the right-hand side of the brain controls the left-hand side of the body and vice versa.

The autonomic nervous system

This controls all those body structures over which we have no conscious control.

The sympathetic system

This system consists of a cord made up of nerve cell bodies. It runs alongside, but outside, the spinal column. It is mainly concerned with the movement of organs such as heart, lungs, pelvic organs, tissues, glandular secretions such as in the skin and the conduction of organ sensations, for example, in the bladder to the spinal cord and brain.

Sympathetic nerves increase and accelerate body activity. They are stimulated by strong emotions, excitement and stress.

The parasympathetic system

This consists mainly of the vagus nerve which supplies organs of the chest and abdomen, but also includes other cranial nerves and some nerves in the lower region of the spinal column.

Like the sympathetic system, the parasympathetic system is concerned with involuntary bodily functions such as secretions of the glands and mucous membranes, muscular movements like digestive peristalsis, and organ sensations.

The parasympathetic system tends to slow down body activity and is particularly concerned with the body's functions during rest.

The sympathetic and parasympathetic divisions of the autonomic nervous system, although opposite, are complementary. Their respective functions are co-ordinated and synchronized to achieve maximum stability of body function during a wide range of daily activities such as reading, eating, running, sleep etc.

Reflex action is a further function of the autonomic nervous system. It is an involuntary reaction to sensory input, e.g. a toddler's recovery of balance to prevent a fall as she learns to walk; removing a body part from extreme cold or heat to prevent damage.

Herbs for the nervous system

Nervines, herbs specific for the nervous system, can be described as 'stimulating the calm', to rebalance our energies and restore physical and emotional equilibrium. In this way nervines defy and transcend classification but offer us their innate harmony.

You will note that several herbs are listed in different categories in the following sections. This is yet again an indication of the dynamic balance that we can achieve through the use of single herbs or their synergistic combinations, depending on our needs.

Nervine tonics

These make a contribution to our well-being and vitality by nourishing and strengthening the nervous system, thereby improving its healthy functioning. They are called for in situations of prolonged stress and exhaustion to ease tension and anxiety, lift depression and restore emotional balance and energy.

Borage	Sage	Vervain
Oats	Skullcap	Wild Betony

Nervine relaxants

These are particularly helpful for people in need of rest, calm and quiet as they are anxious, fearful and tense and often find it difficult to unwind and relax.

Chamomile	Limeflower	Wild Betony
Lavender	Skullcap	Vervain
Lemon Balm	St John's Wort	

Nervine stimulants

Several herbs have an uplifting and invigorating energy, which eases lethargy, debility and depression. Direct nervous stimulation is hardly ever called for, as we tend to suffer from sensory overstimulation.

Borage	Oats	St John's Wort
Lavender	Rosemary	Vervain
Lemon Balm	Skullcap	

Aromatic herbs and spices can also increase general energy and vitality.

Celery	Peppermint
Cinnamon	Sage
Ginger	Thyme

Liver remedies

Should the liver not function effectively in removing toxins and waste products from the bloodstream, these may interfere with the function of the nervous system and lead to headaches, lethargy and depression. The inclusion of bitters will support the body overall.

Burdock root	Marigold
Chamomile	Rosemary
Dandelion root	Vervain

Complaints of the nervous system

All disease, whether physical, emotional or mental, can manifest in the body and must be considered holistically in the context of emotional, mental as well as physical well-being.

A multitude of conditions affect the nervous system and range from predominantly physical problems such as nerve degeneration or damage to a nerve, to emotional manifestations like insomnia, anxiety, stress, to severe emotional and mental health issues.

As the major physical and emotional complaints require professional attention, we will focus on transient conditions that can benefit from self-administered herbs.

Stress

Demands on our physical, emotional and mental energies are part of everyday life and contribute to positive challenges and stimulation. Only when we experience distress from extreme or long-term demands on our energies are we said to suffer from stress.

In this form, stress is a frequent contributing factor in the development of a wide range of diseases since much of our well-being is subject to and/or depends on the smooth functioning of the nervous system.

Conditions significantly influenced by the nervous system can manifest in a number of different bodily systems and are often caused or aggravated by the impact of long-term stress. Most commonly, these are essential hypertension, asthma, skin conditions, various manifestations of indigestion, ulcerative digestive complaints, bowel disorders and glandular imbalances. In order effectively to address these and many other stress-related complaints, a holistic herbal approach will include support for the nervous system. (See suggestions for appropriate treatment in the relevant systems sections.)

Long-term stress, however, can also manifest more directly in complaints associated with the nervous system, notably anxiety, tension, lack of vitality, transient depression and sleeping problems.

Our normal stress response (see also adrenal glands) causes an increase in pulse rate and blood pressure, increased blood supply to the muscles, quickened breathing and the release of glucose from the liver to meet the body's needs for extra energy. During phases of extreme or prolonged stress, the body remains in a state of alertness over an extended period of time. Eventually this will lead to exhaustion of the nervous and circulatory system as well as the adrenal glands, depleting vitality and energy and contributing to ill-health.

While each person reacts differently to demanding situations and experiences stress differently, it is possible to support the body generally as it responds in its individual way.

Our body's nourishment, as stress leaves its marks, needs to be appropriate. Particular attention needs to be paid to sufficient intake of B vitamins and vitamin C in the form of wholegrains and plenty of fresh fruit and vegetables. Stimulants such as sugar, tea, coffee, cigarettes and alcohol should be avoided and the impact of noise and pollution should be appreciated. Gentle exercise, yoga, meditation and relaxation contribute to build quiet and reflective times into our daily routine; these are needed for our physical, emotional and mental well-being.

To find a balance between the multitude of daily demands and the necessary times of peace and tranquillity to give the body an opportunity to recover is of paramount importance. This often needs to be combined with an assessment and re-evaluation of lifestyle.

The regular use of nervine tonics, as they feed and nourish the nervous system, have a prominent role to fulfil in this context.

To tone and strengthen both the nervous system and the adrenal glands and support good liver function I particularly favour a mixture of:

Borage
Oat   in equal parts
Vervain

Tension and anxiety

These are often associated with long-term stress especially as we begin no longer to be able to meet our own or external demands and expectations.

They may manifest in:
- inability to relax and unwind
- muscular tension and cramps
- physical restlessness and agitation
- irritability
- unproductive and fearful thoughts.

Choose from the nervine relaxants as they will all ease tension and anxiety and combine with a suitable nervine tonic.

An uplifting pleasant mixture which can be drunk regularly is:

Peppermint
Vervain   in equal parts

If you suffer especially from fear, try Wood Betony. Anti-spasmodic herbs are useful when there is much muscular tension, especially Chamomile, Lime flower and Lavender. People who do a lot of caring in domestic or professional spheres often benefit from Lemon Balm as it helps to nourish a positive sense of self.

Loss of vitality and depression

Prolonged stress and demands can lead to exhaustion with progressive physical debility, lack of energy and transient depression.

Together with nervine tonics, herbs that have an uplifting and stimulating energy often ease lethargy, debility and depression.

For long-term use, choose from Borage, Vervain, Rosemary and St John's Wort. These combine well with aromatic herbs and spices, which often have a more immediate invigorating effect.

When transient depression is connected with physical loss of vitality and emotional and mental exhaustion, the following teas drunk regularly over a period of time may improve well-being:

Oats   Lemon Balm
Rosemary   **or**   Rosemary
St John's Wort   Vervain
with a pinch of Ginger   in equal parts

For dietary and lifestyle suggestions see above.

Sleeping problems

The lack of restful and deep sleep is often the result of long-term stress and anxiety.

Problems can manifest in different ways with:

■ inability to fall asleep
■ frequent waking during the night
■ waking during the night with inability to go back to sleep
■ disturbing dreams
■ early waking in the morning.

Nervine relaxants such as Chamomile, Lavender or Lime flower will promote restful sleep and can be drunk as a nightcap or a strong infusion can be added to a soothing bath before bed.

If your anxiety leads to fitful sleep with disturbing dreams and thoughts about the demands of the next day, make sure to try Wood Betony with a relaxing nervine such as Lavender or Lemon Balm to help ease your concerns.

Assess your exposure to dietary as well as to environmental stimulants, such as sugar, tea, coffee, alcohol, late meals, loud TV or hectic music. In general, make sure you develop a calm evening routine that allows you to unwind and relax gradually from your day and helps you to focus on your own needs. Make time to have a bath, listen to some music, read or have a pleasant conversation, go for an evening walk.

Headaches

can be caused by a variety of problems. These include:

■ stress and tension
■ increased blood pressure
■ eye disorders
■ hormonal imbalances
■ liver and digestive disorders
■ allergies
■ functional disorders of the nervous system.

For chronic headaches, consult a medical practitioner.

Any of the relaxing herbs may be used to ease a headache, though my favourite mixture is:

Lavender	
Rosemary	in equal parts

The mixture eases muscular tension in neck, shoulders and blood vessels, improving circulation to the head. The mild bitter taste and the calming properties aid the digestion and also make it suitable where headaches are related to digestive disorders.

Migraine

Migraine is a very intense, recurrent headache. It can be associated with nausea and vomiting and be varied in intensity, frequency and duration. Normally it is preceded by visual, motor and mood disturbances.

Migraines tend to be triggered by a range and combination of different factors. Common migraine triggers are:

■ reactions to certain foods:
- coffee
- chocolate
- dairy produce
- alcohol, especially red wine, port, sherry
- chemical food additives
- wheat
- sugar

■ extreme blood sugar fluctuations
■ stress, including flickers from computer/TV screens and artificial lighting
■ hormonal imbalances
■ structural problems in musculoskeletal system.

Treatment involves attention to easing acute attacks as well as discovering and addressing any underlying causes.

For acute attacks, drink at the very earliest indication one cup or 20 drops of tincture in water of:

> Lavender
> Rosemary
> Vervain   in equal parts
>
> Repeat every $^1/_2$ – 1 hour, if needed. Rescue Remedy can also help.

Stop what you are doing immediately and rest. An hour's sleep may well enable you later to carry on with your day.

To address migraines in the long term requires a multifaceted approach:

■ Keep a food diary to help you establish any patterns between your diet and the occurrence of attacks. Exclude any foods you suspect are unsuitable for you and see whether your migraines improve.

■ Explore every aspect of your lifestyle and patterns of exhaustion and stress.

■ Eat regularly; introduce exercise and relaxation into your daily routine; use bitter nervine tonics and relaxants to strengthen the nervous system and support the liver.

■ Assess whether your migraines are related to hormonal fluctuations e.g. during adolescence and the menopause, pre- and/or post-menstrually. (Refer to the section on the Endocrine system for suggestions on hormonal balance.)

■ Consult a cranial osteopath if you feel you may suffer from a structural problem.

Self-treatment of migraines can be difficult. Help from a practitioner may be necessary to tackle such an intransigent problem.

14 | THE ENDOCRINE SYSTEM

Our bodies work efficiently only when the balance in and between all bodily systems as well as organs and cells is monitored, controlled and adjusted. The endocrine system, in close conjunction with the nervous system, helps to maintain our internal environment through hormonal and nervous activity. To be healthy thus requires a well-integrated and balanced endocrine system.

Anatomy and physiology

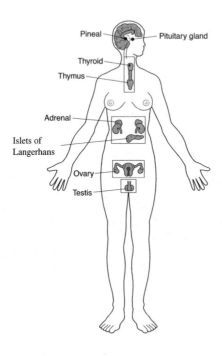

The endocrine system consists of a series of separate but closely related glands that secrete hormones.

Hormones are chemicals that affect cells and organs, usually some distance from their source. The glands secrete their hormones directly into the bloodstream, from which the hormones are circulated all over the body until they reach the target cell or organ. In conjunction with the nervous system, endocrine glands integrate and harmonize the activities of organs and cells by negative and positive feedback mechanisms resulting in growth, reproduction and metabolic stability.

In the liver hormones are converted into inactive compounds and eliminated through the kidneys. Hence hormonal end products can be found and tested for in the urine.

Endocrine tissues and glands are distributed throughout the body and include:

- pituitary gland
- hypothalamus
- thyroid
- parathyroid
- thymus
- pineal gland
- adrenal glands
- sex glands in ovaries and testes
- Islets of Langerhans in pancreas.

Only some of these can be discussed here.

Pituitary gland

The pituitary gland is the main gland involved in endocrine function. It consists of a frontal and rear lobe. Many hormones are secreted by the frontal lobe, including growth hormones, male and female sex hormones, and hormones that regulate the thyroid and the adrenal cortex as well as metabolic hormones.

The rear lobe produces oxytocin, which causes uterine contractions during birth, and vasopressin, which promotes water absorption from the kidneys and influences blood pressure.

Hypothalamus

The hypothalamus, a collection of nerve cells forming the control centre of the sympathetic and parasympathetic nervous system, releases hormones to the pituitary gland. Through the pituitary it is involved in the metabolism of fat, carbohydrate and water and with sleep, body temperature and sexual functions.

Thyroid

The thyroid secretes iodine-containing hormones that control general metabolism.

Adrenal glands

The adrenal glands lie over each kidney and are divided into an inner (medulla) and outer (cortex) part.

The outer part produces cortico-steroids involved in the control of sodium/potassium balance, storage of glucose and the production of sex hormones. The outer part of the adrenal glands acts in response to stimulation from the pituitary hormones. Any weakness in function of either gland will have repercussions on the secretion of the other and hence overall well-being. Often it is beneficial to support both glands herbally at the same time.

In contrast, the inner part of the adrenals respond to stressful situations, pain, extremes of temperature, emotional shock etc., which trigger the 'flight or fight' mechanism. The hypothalamus will be stimulated to transmit impulses that will release adrenalin and noradrenalin into the bloodstream activating breathing, pulse rate and heart function as well as increasing the blood pressure in anticipation of extreme physical and mental activity. Glucose is also released from the liver to meet the need for increased energy. This mechanism will take place regardless of the type of stress involved.

Islets of Langerhans

The Islets of Langerhans in the pancreas secrete insulin which regulates the blood sugar and the conversion of sugars into heat and energy.

Herbs for the endocrine system

Endocrine tonics

These help to promote the healthy functions of the endocrine system and to regulate overall hormonal balance. They combine well with nervine tonics to improve hormonal and emotional balance in long-term stress and ill-health.

Borage
Oats

Pituitary gland balancers

These help to regulate, through either stimulation or inhibition, the production of pituitary gland hormones. Reproductive problems due to hormonal imbalances often benefit from these balancers:

Sage
Chaste Tree berries

Adrenal gland tonics

These help to promote the functions of the adrenal gland and to regulate the production of adrenal hormones; they are particularly relevant in times of prolonged ill-health and stress.

Borage
Ginger
Liquorice root

Adrenal gland stimulants

These increase the production of adrenal hormones.

Celery seed	Rosemary
Liquorice root	Thyme
Nettle	

Adrenal gland relaxants

These inhibit the production of adrenal hormones, particularly through general relaxation, and combine well with relaxing nervine tonics.

Vervain

Bitter herbs and alteratives

These are also helpful in the treatment of the endocrine system as they holistically cleanse, tone and stimulate the body and promote overall well-being.

Complaints of the endocrine system

Causes of problems in the endocrine system range from external factors such as long-term emotional and physical stress to tumours and genetic disorders. Here we will focus on minor complaints, which lend themselves to self-treatment with herbs.

The herbal approach encompasses the use of herbs specific to the functions of different glands, improvement of overall well-being and vitality as well as dietary suggestions.

Pituitary imbalance

Even minor malfunction of the pituitary gland can lead to diverse complaints, most noticeably those related to the reproductive system.

Chaste Tree is known to help balance the functions of the pituitary gland, especially the secretion of female and male sex hormones (see reproductive system), whereas *Sage* is particularly benefical to women's reproductive health. Both herbs work particularly effectively when combined with restorative endocrine tonics.

Watercress is nutritive to the pituitary gland and restorative to its balance and should actively be included in one's diet in salads, soups and juices.

Supplementation with Evening Primrose or Borage oil may also help to restore balanced function.

Adrenal exhaustion

Any form of prolonged stress will eventually lead to exhaustion of the adrenal glands and the nervous system. Other bodily systems frequently involved are the circulation and heart, liver and lungs.

In order actively to prevent adrenal exhaustion, if living a hectic lifestyle with long-term stresses, care should be taken to avoid all stimulants such as sugar, coffee, tea, alcohol and cigarettes as they compound the effects of adrenalin and noradrenalin and lead to further exhaustion.

Instead, a well-balanced diet rich in fruit and vegetables, especially watercress and varied nuts, seeds and wholegrains for the B vitamin will help to maintain well-being and vitality. Eating regularly helps to avoid excessive blood sugar fluctuations and their attendant drop in energy levels, lack of concentration, irritability and sugar cravings.

One or two cups of Rosemary tea daily sweetened with a little honey can be drunk regularly in order to maintain energy levels and concentration.

Should high stress levels lead to agitation, anxiety and exhaustion, Vervain tea helps to balance mental and physical energies and restore intellectual clarity.

Should a tonic be called for, Borage tea drunk regularly is an effective revitalizer of the adrenal glands, especially of the inner part, whereas Liquorice is indicated in rebalancing the function of the gland's outer part. These can be combined according to need.

A pleasant restorative infusion which can be drunk regularly is the following:

Borage
Oats
Vervain   in equal parts
with a pinch of Ginger

The long-term health and function of the immune system is also mediated by the health of the adrenal glands and will be negatively affected by any weakness (see also immune system).

15 | THE SKIN

The skin protects us against external micro-organisms and injury, from sunlight and the extremes of temperature. A stable internal environment is maintained by the skin through preserving water, salt and organic substances in the body while excreting waste products in liaison with kidneys, bowel and the lungs.

The skin also mirrors our health and age. Many signs indicative of our physical or emotional well-being are reflected in the skin such as colour, when lacking regular fresh air and outdoor exercise, dryness with advancing age, pallor and flushing of infectious conditions with fever, blushing with embarrassment and clamminess of hands when nervous.

Equally important, through its rich supply of sensory cells and nerves, the skin enables us to be in physical contact with our external environment, indicating the close interrelationship between the nervous system, the skin and the environment.

As the skin reflects internal problems and imbalances as well as our emotional well-being and our relationships with the outer world, diseases of the skin need to be treated in their entire complexity.

Anatomy and physiology

The skin, the largest and also a complex organ of the body, holds a number of different functions as it:
- protects the whole body
- provides a physical barrier against injury, the invasion of foreign substances and ultra-violet sunrays
- regulates temperature
- is a sensory receptor

■ eliminates water, salt and waste-products
■ synthesizes vitamin D.

The skin is divided into two parts:

■ The epidermis, the outer part, has a number of different layers. The outermost is made up of dehydrated cells, which are continuously cast off as scales.
■ The dermis, or true skin, consists of connective tissue and contains:
  – the blood and lymphatic system, which provides a very fine and dense network of blood and lymphatic vessels
  – a fat layer, beneath the dermis, which functions as a shock absorber and conserver of body heat
  – sensory receptors and nerves, which react to pain, heat/cold, pressure and itching and contribute to the regulation of body temperature
  – sweat glands, which are responsible for the elimination of water, salt and waste products and are also involved in the regulation of body temperature

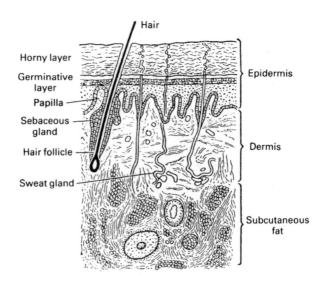

- sebaceous glands secrete sebum, which is primarily composed of fats.

In addition skin also consists of muscles, hair follicles and a variety of cells, chemicals and bacteria. Nails are outgrowths from the epidermis.

Herbs for the skin

Vulneraries

These are herbs that facilitate the healing of tissues and can be used internally and externally. Depending on need, choose from vulneraries that are more emollient or demulcent, or those with a more astringent action.

Agrimony	Ribwort
Comfrey	Yarrow
Marigold	

Anti-microbials

These may be called for to aid the skin in dealing with invading micro-organisms.

Echinacea	Marigold
Garlic	Thyme
Lavender	

Alteratives

These deeply cleanse and detoxify the whole body. Common alteratives used in the treatment of skin complaints are.

Burdock root	Nettle
Cleavers	Red Clover
Marigold	

Diaphoretics

These aid the skin in eliminating toxins as they improve the blood supply to the surface of the skin and increase sweating. Some will also generally stimulate the circulation:

| Ginger | Rosemary |
| Lime flower | Yarrow |

Diuretics

These have an important role to play in the treatment of skin complaints as they facilitate the elimination of waste through the urinary system.

| Cleavers | Nettle |
| Dandelion leaf | Yarrow |

Nervines

These help to restore our physical and emotional balance. Given the close connection between healthy skin and our emotional well-being, nervine tonics and relaxants make a valuable contribution to the treatment of skin complaints.

Chamomile	Skullcap
Lavender	Vervain
Lemon Balm	Wood Betony

Complaints of the skin

The protective and eliminative functions of the skin, its extensive network of blood and lymph vessels and the close relationship with the nervous system are reflected in many skin conditions.

Eczema

The term eczema or dermatitis tends to include a wide variety of skin conditions, all of which have the following features in common:

- Skin is itchy, red and inflamed.
- Abrasions are frequent on elbows, back of the knees, wrists, ankles and the face, although eczema may manifest anywhere on the body.
- Eczema may start with minute blisters which fill with colourless fluid. On bursting they leave a weepy rash that can lead to bleeding or cracked and scaly skin.

■ Alternatively, the rash may be red, scaly and very dry and, if the problem is prolonged, the skin may harden, thicken and easily crack and bleed.

■ Scratching may introduce micro-organisms, followed by infections.

Eczema is essentially an allergic condition. Often there is an inherited susceptibility, but also nutritional deficiencies of essential fatty acids, zinc, B 12, calcium and magnesium may play an important role in its development.

It commonly, but not exclusively, starts in babyhood with the introduction of milk formula and/or solid foods; subsequently asthma and hay fever may also manifest. An allergic reaction to substances that we frequently touch – metals, detergents, fabrics – is also a common cause. As eczema tends to be closely linked to our emotional well-being, its appearance may fluctuate and disappear for many months and even years to recur when we are low in vitality and emotionally and physically unwell or exhausted. Not uncommonly, eczema may also be brought to light in later life by stress, exhaustion and emotional upset.

It is essential to establish the cause of eczema and any contributing factors as far as possible so that it can be treated holistically.

A useful basic mixture can be prepared by using:

Borage	
Burdock root	
Nettle	
Red Clover or Marigold	
Vervain	in equal parts

This mixture aids the digestive processes, the liver and kidneys, cleanses the lymphatic system, supports the nervous system, adrenal glands and generally nourishes physical and emotional well-being.

Compresses can be cooling and soothing and help to reduce itching and inflammation as well as healing infections and cracks in the skin.

Use singly or in combination:

Chamomile
Comfrey
Marigold

Alternatively, creams with the same herbs can be used where the skin is weepy, whereas ointments are more suitable where dryness of the skin is a marked feature.

To reduce the burden on the immune system challenging foods should be strictly avoided. These most commonly are:

■ cow's milk dairy products
■ wheat
■ eggs

but may also include:

■ citrus fruit
■ tomatoes
■ peppers and aubergine
■ sugar
■ chocolate
■ artificial additives.

To aid the cleansing process, plenty of liquid should be drunk in the form of water, real fruit juices and herb teas, and fresh fruit and vegetables should form a major part of the diet. Make sure to include unrefined oils in the diet such as Linseed, Sunflower and olive oil, pulses, nuts, seeds and fatty fish, if appropriate. For long-term nutritional support, an Evening Primrose oil supplement may prove invaluable to the immune system.

Certain situations can aggravate eczema and should be avoided:

■ Water can irritate and be drying to the skin, especially if chlorinated. Add a teaspoon of vegetable oil to your bath water and moisturize skin after a bath, shower or swimming.
■ Synthetic materials and wool next to the skin may aggravate the condition, as they tend to irritate the skin and increase sweating.
■ Avoid soaps and detergents.
■ If your eczema flares up in the cold, support your circulation with regular exercise and appropriate herbs.

■ If your eczema worsens with stress and anxiety, avoid coffee, tea, alcohol and sugar and follow guidelines on how to deal with stress (see Nervous system).

Acne

Acne is a common feature of adolescence caused by the hormonal changes and increased activity of sebaceous glands as well as the body's ability to metabolize fat and carbohydrates during this time.

Acne manifests with:

■ pustules and cysts, especially on the face, neck and chest
■ a worsening pre-menstrually in young women
■ an improvement in the summer and worsening in the winter.

A cleansing mixture such as:

Burdock root Dandelion root Nettle Red Clover   in equal parts Echinacea may be needed, if extensive infections are causing concern.

The dietary intake of fruits, vegetables and fluids needs to be encouraged while fats, sweets and carbohydrates need to be reduced. Low zinc levels are often noted and can be remedied with supplements.

Meticulous hygiene supported with the frequent use of a lotion of equal parts of distilled Witch Hazel and Rosewater with Marigold helps to tone, heal and astringe overactive skin glands and pores.

Heat rash or Prickly heat

This is an inflammation of the skin. It manifests with:
■ an itchy rash of red or pink spots, commonly raised and found on the trunk, shoulders, arms and neck
■ is aggravated by sweating

■ scratching can lead to possible invasion of staphylococci and subsequent infection.

To cool the skin, shower or bath frequently with tepid water. To help reduce inflammation and itching add Chamomile or Marigold to the water or use a strong tea as a rinse:

Chamomile	
Nettle	
Peppermint	in equal parts

Such tea drunk warm throughout the day helps to remove excess heat from the body, reduces itching and soothes irritated skin.

As heat rash can be an indication of a toxic overload or an excessively 'hot' diet avoid any foods which cause sweating such as hot drinks, peppery spices such as cayenne, onion and garlic, reduce your meat and dairy produce intake and increase fresh fruits, vegetables and salads. Drink plenty of water.

Cold sores

Cold sores are caused by the herpes simplex virus and frequently develop when we are emotionally and/or physically run-down.

Common symptoms are:

■ small blisters especially around the mouth, which ulcerate and form a scab

■ a slight fever

■ lymph glands in the neck may be swollen.

Herbal treatment aims at aiding the immune system and improving eliminative function through the use of alteratives and lymphatic cleansers. Lemon balm is said to be specific against the virus:

Lemon Balm	
Echinacea	
Marigold	in equal parts
Drink frequently until healing is complete.	

To aid the healing process and limit the spreading of the infection, apply any of the following directly to any sores:

Echinacea
Marigold
Lavender
Lemon Balm

Avoid touching or scratching the sores. In the case of children ensure that they have clean hands and well-cut fingernails to help prevent the spread of the infection. For the same reason, keep your towels etc. separate. Drink plenty of fluid and eat raw vegetables and fruit.

Wounds

Marigold is the choice herb for cuts and abrasions.

Comfrey, too, is a respected wound healer as it promotes cell proliferation and granulation of tissue especially important in broken bones. Both plants can be used as a poultice, a compress, a strong tea or in creams and ointments.

The healing and astringent properties of *Ribwort* often come into their own when we need something immediately. The fresh leaf widely available in both urban and rural settings can be applied directly to the wound to staunch bleeding and help the healing process. If there is any danger of infection, *Echinacea* should be added to any preparation.

An infusion of *Chamomile* or *Lavender* counteracts shock and settles agitation resulting from accident. At the same time a soothing tea provides needed fluid as dehydration delays wound healing.

Part III
The herbal

Forty-five herbs are explored and listed in alphabetical order of their common English names.

Each plant has been chosen according to the following criteria:

- The herb by itself has a wide range of comprehensive healing properties.
- The herb has synergistic compatibility with the other herbs selected.
- The herb is easily available locally as it is part of the Western European flora or a commonly used spice.
- The herb is generally safe to use.
- The total of the herbs listed fulfils most of our day-to-day health needs.

The information about each herb is presented within the following format:

- **Common name** of the herb.
- **Latin name**, plant family.
- **Part used**: part of the plant used medicinally is given.
- **Constituents**: The most relevant (or known) chemical components of the plant are listed in order of priority; if required, refer to Part I for more information, especially on chemistry and pharmacology.
- **Actions**: A list of the most relevant actions of the herb is given in order of priority. Refer to Appendix 1.
- **Uses**: Historical and contemporary uses of the herb are described with reference to different complaints; the qualities and energies are mentioned where appropriate.

■ **Dosage**: Quantities for the use of standard infusions or decoctions and tinctures are given, based on standard adult quantities per single dosage; refer Chapter 18 for more information on dosage, especially for children and the elderly.

■ **Cautions**: Listed where appropriate.

For ease of reference also included here is a list of actions of herbs together with brief explanations as well as guidelines on dosages for different ages and herbs contra-indicated in pregnancy. The section on intuitive work with herbs is envisaged to help complement and expand the information offered in the herbal with your own personal experiences.

The herbal can help to identify herbs relevant to specific complaints or patterns of diseases and should be used to study herbs mentioned in Part II and the repertory. It also serves as a reference section for further independent study.

16 | HERBS A-Z

Agrimony

Agrimonia eupatoria, Rosaceae

Part used: Aerial.

Constituents: Tannins, bitter principles, volatile oil, vitamins B, K, silica, iron.

Actions: Astringent, diuretic, bitter tonic.

Uses: Agrimony's established reputation as a popular medicinal herb is based on the combination of astringency and bitter properties. As a mild tonic and astringent it is indicated in both acute and chronic conditions.

Agrimony can be used effectively in diarrhoea, kidney and bladder irritation, gastric ulcers and is of particular importance in the treatment of appendicitis.

The bitter components stimulate digestive and liver secretions, making Agrimony a useful remedy in chronic indigestion as a result of liver and gall bladder weakness. Due to the plant's high silica content it relieves sore throats and laryngitis when used as a gargle and will heal wounds and bruises when applied externally.

Dosage: Infusion 8–16 g.
Tincture: 1–5 ml.

Caution: Avoid long-term use with constipation.

Bearberry

Arctostaphylos uva-ursi, Ericaceae

Part used: Leaves.

Constituents: Tannins, flavonoids acids, resin, minerals, trace elements.

Actions: urinary antiseptic, diuretic, astringent.

Uses: The uses of this plant are very specific as Bearberry has drying and cooling qualities with antiseptic and astringent actions on the mucous membranes that make it especially helpful in the treatment of acute urinary infections. Bearberry will soothe, tone and strengthen kidneys and bladder in conditions with frequent, urgent and painful micturition and blood in the urine such as cystitis, urethritis and prostatitis. It combines well with a demulcent when treating these conditions.

For chronic conditions, Bearberry works best with diuretics such as Dandelion leaves or Nettle that help to flush out the urinary system.

Dosage: Infusion 4–8 g.
          Tincture: 1–4 ml.

Caution: Do not take Bearberry on its own for more than a few days as its high tannin content may upset the digestion.

Borage

Borago officinalis, Boraginaceae

Part used: leaf, flower, seed.

Constituents: Mucilage, tannins, saponins, volatile oil, potassium, calcium.

Actions: Demulcent, diuretic, anti-depressive, adrenal gland restorative, expectorant, galactagogue, emollient.

Uses: Throughout history Borage has been used to strengthen the heart, lift depression and dispel melancholy. It also has been valued to promote breast milk and regulate the menstrual cycle. These uses are explained by the restorative action exerted on the adrenal glands when used as a tonic over a period of time.

Long-term stress, mental and nervous exhaustion and general depletion after treatment with steroids (e.g. cortisones) respond well to the strengthening effects of Borage. Hormonal fluctuations during adolescence, pre-menstrually and during the menopause can be eased with Borage due to the stimulation of prostaglandins. During the Middle Ages Borage was a much respected heart remedy,, specifically for palpitations, anxiety and depression. Its anti-inflammatory and demulcent properties help in the cases of hot digestive and respiratory inflammations such as gastritis, colitis, pleurisy and bronchitis.The infusion of the leaves and flowers is soothing and cooling in fevers as well as detoxifying.The young leaves eaten raw taste of cucumber and make a refreshing addition to salads.

Borage oil, prepared from the seeds, contains important fatty acids.

Dosage: Infusion 8–14 g.

Tincture: 2–5 ml.

Burdock

Arctium lappa, Compositae

Part used: Root.

Constituents: bitter glycosides, mucilage, tannins, various acids, inulin, vitamins A, B, C, minerals, especially iron and sulphur.

Actions: Alterative, diuretic, bitter, laxative.

Uses: Burdock is a potent blood cleanser and alterative, useful in all conditions of long-term disharmony that manifest in skin complaints, such as eczema, psoriasis and boils, swollen glands, muscle and joint pain and abdominal congestion. Dioscorides described the internal and external use of the root for both toxic conditions and old sores. Burdock stimulates liver and gall bladder function and, like other alteratives, shifts waste from the cells and tissues into the bloodstream. Care should therefore be taken to support urinary elimination with a nourishing diuretic such as Nettle or Cleavers.

Burdock's purifying and harmonizing potential is best appreciated when taken over a period of time whereby it also strengthens immune function in allergic conditions. In skin conditions,

Burdock's internal use is best complemented with external applications of compresses, creams or ointments for which the fresh leaves can be used. The infused oil has a long-standing reputation for relieving scalp and hair conditions such as dandruff, itchy scalp and loss of hair. As a massage oil it eases hot muscle and joint pains.

Dosage: Decoction: 6–12 g.
            Tincture: 1–5 ml.

Chamomile

Matricaria chamomilla, Compositae

Part used: Flowers.

Constituents: Volatile oils, flavonoids, coumarins, bitter glycosides, tannins.

Actions: Anti-spasmodic, carminative, anti-inflammatory, analgesic, antiseptic, bitter, emetic, vulnerary.

Uses: Chamomile, due to its profoundly balancing nature, is probably one of the most effective herbs to address a wide range of common minor ailments at both acute and chronic levels. Its taste is sweetly aromatic and slightly bitter and in effect balancing to the temperatures of different conditions.

Essentially, Chamomile is a relaxing herb with particular affinity for the digestive and nervous system, although menstrual, respiratory, skin and inflammatory conditions all benefit from it, as it addresses a wide variety of conditions caused or aggravated by tension.

In the nervous system, Chamomile subdues nerve irritability and pain as much as it eases emotional tension and agitation. It is helpful in headaches, insomnia, mood swings, neuralgic pains, infant teething and menstrual discomforts.

In the gastro-intestinal and respiratory tracts, Chamomile reduces irritation and inflammation of the mucous membranes, whereby it exerts a calming and healing influence. People with gastric ulcers, irritable bowels and chronic constipation as well as coughs, sinusitis, hay fever and asthma are likely to benefit from Chamomile.

As a diaphoretic, Chamomile is useful at the onset of colds, flu and fevers, especially those due to children's infectious diseases. A pleasant inhalation can be prepared from the flowers to ease bronchial and sinus conditions.

Irritating itchy and inflamed skin complaints such as mouth ulcers, eczema, nettle rash, heat rash, wounds and sunburn respond well to both internal and external use of Chamomile. Cold or hot infusions for washes or additions to a bath, compresses and ointments make effective external applications.

Dosage: Infusion: 6–14 g.
Tincture: 3–5 ml.

Celery seed

Apium graveolens, Umbelliferae

Part used: Seed.

Constituents: Volatile oils, flavonoids, vitamins A, B, C, E, minerals, trace elements.

Actions: Diuretic, anti-rheumatic, urinary antiseptic, carminative, galactagogue.

Uses: Celery seed finds its main use in chronic toxic conditions which frequently manifest with joint pains and stiffness, muscular aches and swellings such as arthritis, rheumatism and gout.

Mental exhaustion, fatigue and depression, so often associated with chronic pain and discomfort greatly benefit from the nourishing and restoring qualities of Celery seed as it also strengthens adrenal weakness and a depleted nervous system.

The antiseptic and diuretic properties also make Celery an important remedy for acute urinary infections and chronic urinary discomfort.

As a herb which calms and soothes the digestion, Celery can be used to relieve wind, nausea and indigestion. Like Fennel, it is useful for breast-feeding mothers and their babies as it stimulates the flow of breast milk while easing infant colic.

Dosage: Decoction: 8–10 g.
Tincture: 2–5 ml.

Caution: Avoid in pregnancy and with organic kidney disease.

Chaste Tree

Vitex agnus-castus, Verbenaceae

Part used: Berries.

Constituents: Volatile oils, glycosides, bitters, flavonoids.

Actions: Galactagogue, reproductive tonic, hormone regulator, relaxant, diuretic.

Uses: Throughout history the berries have been used to harmonize and balance reproductive functions in both women and men. Modern research indicates that it stimulates and balances the functions of the pituitary gland, particularly in relation to female sex hormones and the reduction of prolactin secretions. Through its overall balancing effects on hormone levels, it normalizes the balance of the sex hormone, and appears to support the production hormone especially in the second half of the menstrual cycle.

Due to the effect of the berries on regulating hormones, they hold a central place in the treatment of hormone-related gynaecological conditions. It is the remedy of choice in addressing pre-menstrual complaints, irregular or heavy periods, fibroids and fibro-cystic breast changes. Chaste Tree will also help to stimulate fertility and can prevent early miscarriages when due to hormonal difficulties. In nursing mothers it will stimulate the production of breast milk. After child birth or breast feeding as well as after the use of the contraceptive pill, Chaste Tree can help to reestablish a healthy hormonal balance, easing mood swings and physical discomforts.

During the menopause, it can be taken to ease such common symptoms as hot flushes, night sweats, low vitality, vaginal dryness, sleep disturbances and depression.

During puberty, Chaste Tree can clear up acne in both young women and men if it is related to hormone fluctuations and sluggish liver function.

Although Chaste Tree is mostly considered these days to be a woman's remedy, the ancients valued it equally in addressing male sexual functions and used it to treat male impotence, premature ejaculation and spermatorrhoea.

As the pituitary gland is at its most active in the morning, Chaste Tree is best taken on rising before breakfast. It has a spicy, pungent and slightly bitter taste with a warming and stimulating energy. Take regularly for 4–6 months and then phase out gradually by reducing the dosage. For best results and where appropriate, Chaste Tree should be complemented by other remedies such as adrenal, liver and gynaecological tonics.

Dosage: Infusion: 4–10 g 1 x day on rising.
Tincture: 10–20 drops 1 x day on rising.

Caution: Use under professional guidance during pregnancy and while breast feeding.

Cinnamon

Cinnamomum zeylandicum or cassia, Lauraceae

Part used: Bark.

Constituents: Volatile oils, tannins, mucilage, resin.

Actions: Anti-microbial, carminative, anti-spasmodic, astringent.

Uses: Cinnamon bark is a sweet and aromatic stimulant with warming, carminative and astringent qualities. The sweet taste is favoured by children and adults alike.

When the decoction is drunk hot, the stimulating effect on the heart and circulation is profound, dispelling any cold and flu symptoms and rapidly warming cold extremities. The strongly anti-microbial volatile oil at the same time helps to reduce infections in the respiratory and digestive systems.

In digestive complaints, Cinnamon is best enjoyed warm, whereby its warming and stimulating qualities will relieve complaints due to cold and muscular tension. This makes it a pleasant and effective remedy for nausea, vomiting, flatulence, colic and acute and chronic diarrhoea, including dysentery.

Cinnamon is also successfully used to check heavy menstrual bleeding when accompanied by pelvic congestion and poor uterine muscle tone. In conjunction with other remedies, Cinnamon can therefore be useful in the treatment of fibroids and endometriosis.

Small quantities taken over a period of time will correct poor circulation manifesting as cold hands and feet and boost energy and vitality.

Dosage: Decoction: 2–5 g.
Tincture: 0.2–2 ml.

Caution: Avoid in hot conditions, contra-indicated in pregnancy and while breast feeding.

Cleavers

Galium aparine, Rubiaceae

Part used: Aerial.

Constituents: Coumarins, tannins, citric and gallitannic acids, saponins, trace elements.

Actions: Alterative, diuretic, astringent, nutritive.

Uses: A potent lymphatic tonic, Cleavers alters the blood and fluid environment, increasing the elimination of waste products and toxins.

By drawing on its alterative and diuretic actions, Cleavers, traditionally used as part of a spring tonic, benefits people with chronic lymphatic disorders such as swollen glands, tonsillitis and adenoid problems and dry, itchy skin complaints such as dry eczema and psoriasis.

Cleavers can also be used as a soothing urinary remedy in the treatment of acute infections such as cystitis and prostatitis combining its cooling energy with demulcent and astringent properties.

Externally, compresses and lotions can be applied to cool and soothe skin inflammations and sunburn.

Cleavers make an excellent nourishing vegetable and a cooling and energizing juice.

Dosage: Infusion: 8–16 g.
Tincture: 2–5 ml.

Comfrey

Symphytum officinale, Boraginaceae

Part used: Root, leaf.

Constituents: mucilage, tannins, alkaloids, allantoin, inulin, steroidal saponins, volatile oils, resin, vitamins A, B12, C, E, minerals, trace elements.

Actions: Astringent, demulcent, expectorant, vulnerary.

Uses: Comfrey is the prime remedy for wound healing.

Internally, it can be used for hot, dry conditions of mucous membrane irritation. The high mucilage content combined with tannins soothes, protects and heals inflamed and hot tissues, especially helpful in gastritis, colitis and peptic ulcers as well as dry coughs, laryngitis and bronchitis. Likewise, externally, Comfrey will heal burns, bruises and cuts. Care should be taken, however, when treating deep wounds. Hildegard von Bingen observed the possible problem of abscess formation due to superficial skin healing. Ensure the wound is well cleaned and combine Comfrey with antiseptic wound healers such as Marigold, Ribwort or St John's Wort.

The high allantoin content makes Comfrey a specific for bone fractures and promotes speedy recovery. Internal use and external application in the form of a poultice, compress or ointment is recommended.

Comfrey leaf has long been valued as a nourishing vegetable rich in minerals, vitamins, especially B12, and trace elements. Comfrey nourishes the blood and improves anaemia, fatigue and general weakness due to nutritional deficiencies.

Emotionally, Comfrey is helpful to those who lack grounding and boundaries. It gradually builds up a solid foundation and lends structure, stamina and emotional focus to one's intentions.

Dosage: Infusion/decoction: 6–16 g.
Tincture: 2–4 ml.

Caution: Comfrey leaf only is recommended for long-term internal use.

Cramp Bark

Viburnum opulus, Caprifoliaceae

Part used: Bark.

Constituents: Bitter, valerianic acid, salicylates, resin, tannin.

Actions: Anti-spasmodic, sedative, astringent.

Uses: As the name suggests, Cramp Bark is an anti-spasmodic herb, used to relieve muscular tension and spasm. Its application ranges from painful cramps in the legs and lower back pain, muscular bladder irritation to tension in the lower respiratory system and heart palpitations due to stress. Most specifically though, Cramp Bark is used as a women's remedy for a range of painful gynaecological conditions especially during menstruation and ovulation. As a herb that eases uterine tension as well as relieving uterine congestion, Cramp Bark is effective in spasmodic dysmenorrhea with cramping before the onset and congestive dysmenorrhea with dragging pains in the lower pelvis and slowly developing bleeding. Its additional astringent quality makes it useful in heavy bleeding, especially when associated with the menopause.

Dosage: Decoction: 8–14 g.
          Tincture: 2–5 ml.

Dandelion

Taraxacum officinale, Compositae

Part used: Root, leaf.

Constituents: Bitter glycosides, resin, volatile oils, tannins, acids, vitamins A, C, minerals especially potassium.

Actions: bitter tonic, diuretic, laxative, detoxifying, nutrient.

Uses: *Root*: Dandelion root is probably the most frequently used digestive bitter remedy with slight laxative, diuretic and alterative actions.

Its bitter taste stimulates saliva, digestive and pancreatic enzymes, gastric juices and bile. It is effective in conditions associated with congestion of the liver and gall bladder. These include hepatitis, jaundice, inflammation of the gall bladder, sluggish bowels and indigestion as well as haemorrhoids and varicose veins. Additional diuretic and alterative effects make the root important in the treatment of arthritic and rheumatic conditions, chronic skin complaints such as eczema and herpes and a general tendency to infections. When taken long-term, the root promotes overall detoxification. The root's high inulin content, especially when collected in the autumn, improves pancreatic functions and can be beneficial in the control of blood sugar levels in response to carbohydrates.

I have also used the root effectively in dispelling hot fiery emotions manifesting in, for example, physical and mental hyperactivity and insomnia. The cooling and grounding effects of the root together with its detoxifying actions harmonize physical and emotional energies allowing for a balanced well-being.

Leaf: Dandelion leaf is similar in constituents to the root, although less bitter, but more strongly diuretic with a high potassium content.

Dandelion leaf is mainly used as a potent diuretic in all conditions characterized by water retention. Traditionally, it was included in spring tonics, together with Nettle and Cleavers, and the young leaves are excellent when eaten fresh in salads or prepared as a juice.

Dosage: *Leaf*: Infusion 8–16g.
       Root: Decoction 6–16 g.
       Tincture: 2–5 ml.

Echinacea

Echinacea angustifolia, Compositae

Part used: Root, whole plant.

Constituents: Volatile oils, glycosides, tannins, resins, vitamin C, trace elements.

Action: Anti-microbial, alterative.

Uses: Echinacea is a North American plant that was extensively used in Native American healing before being incorporated into herbal use by white settlers. Over the last few years Echinacea has become increasingly popular in Europe. It is commonly perceived, and marketed, as an immune enhancer to be taken long-term to stimulate immune function and reduce infections.

Echinacea temporarily stimulates the body's defence system and its activities and enhances the body's abilities to address microbial infections. Its immediate efficacy in stimulating immune functions is particularly noticable when exposed to potential infections such as during an outbreak of cold, flu, typhoid and the various childhood infections. During such times a short – say, 10-day – course of Echinacea is very effective in supporting and strengthening the body. In cases of infection, Echinacea is likely to reduce the severity and length of illness.

Used long term, Echinacea is an effective alterative and lymphatic cleanser, especially valuable in the treatment of chronic inflammations such as acne, boils, abscesses, swollen lymph glands and chronic catarrhal complaints.

Applied externally, as lotion, compress or in creams and ointments, Echinacea's anti-microbial action promotes healing of infected wounds and skin ulcers. Douches can be used to arrest vaginal discharges.

Dosage: Decoction: 6–10 g.
           Tincture: 2–4 ml.

Caution: The overall stimulating effect of the plant can at times cause dizziness and nausea, especially when taken in large quantities. In my experience, small but frequent dosages tend to be more effective particularly in acute conditions.

Elderflower

Sambucus nigra, Caprifoliaceae

Part used: Flowers.

Constituents: Flavonoids, volatile oils, glycosides, tannin.

Actions: Diaphoretic, diuretic, expectorant, emollient.

Uses: Although many parts of the Elder tree were used medicinally – the flowers, leaves, berries, bark, root and young shoots, the flowers are best known for their medicinal properties. With their sweet taste and uplifting energy, they are also the most versatile. Elderflowers are predominantly used for those respiratory complaints associated with excessive catarrh, both chronic and acute. An infusion can be used with great effect in colds, sinus problems, sore throats, tonsillitis, laryngitis, coughs with excessive phlegm, etc. Taken long term, Elderflowers restore the mucous membranes of the respiratory system and balance mucus secretions. Thus it is an important remedy in hay fever, allergic rhinitis, chronic sinusitis and asthma.

The flowers are sweat inducing especially when taken as a hot infusion. It is an excellent remedy to lower fevers in colds, flu and children's infectious diseases.

Through its diuretic action, Elderflower positively influences the fluid balance of the body and can be used for water retention, urinary sluggishness and deposits.

Elderflowers are light, expansive and uplifting in energy. They can be used to shift emotional stagnation and blocked creativity.

Dosage: Infusion: 6–14 g.
Tincture: 2–4 ml.

Fennel

Foeniculum vulgare, Umbelliferae

Part used: Seeds.

Constituents: Volatile oils, fixed oils, flavonoids, coumarins, silica.

Actions: Anti-spasmodic, carminative, expectorant, diuretic, galactagogue.

Uses: Fennel, strongly aromatic and deeply warming and balancing, is best known for its ability to calm and soothe the digestion. Its reputation as a remedy for flatulence, indigestion, nausea and vomiting goes back to ancient Egyptian times and is still relevant today. Hildegard von Bingen advocates the regular use of Fennel after meals to balance the digestion, improve eyesight and ensure well-being and joyfulness. This approach is reflected in the Indian custom of chewing Fennel seeds after meals.

Coughs, bronchitis and wheezing also benefit from the warming, anti-spasmodic and demulcent properties, which relax respiratory tension and ease expectoration.

As a diuretic, Fennel can be used to relieve water retention and urinary irritation. It therefore is helpful in arthritis, bladder complaints, bed wetting and incontinence. Breast-feeding mothers could hardly find a more suitable drink than Fennel tea as it ensures a regular supply of breast milk while at the same time dispelling digestive unease and wind in a colicky baby.

With its gentle oestrogenic action and warming and stimulating quality, Fennel eases menstrual conditions characterized by poor pelvic circulation, cramps, scanty flow, blood clots and premenstrual water retention.

Dosage: Decoction: 6–12g.
Tincture: 2–4 ml.

Caution: Avoid in pregnancy.

Garlic

Allium sativum, Liliaceae

Part used: Bulb.

Constituents: Volatile oils, sulphurous components, vitamins A, B, C, trace elements.

Actions: Anti-microbial, diaphoretic, anti-spasmodic, expectorant, hypotensive, anti-coagulant, anthelmintic.

Uses: Garlic has been a respected remedy around the globe for thousands of years. It is one of the most effective anti-microbials with anti-bacterial, anti-viral, anti-fungal and anti-parasitic actions exerted throughout the body.

Garlic can be used for bronchial and lung infections, colds, sinusitis, flu, etc. The additional stimulating and decongesting properties help to clear catarrh and make Garlic a potent expectorant for acute or chronic bronchitis, whooping cough and congested lungs. By promoting sweating, Garlic helps to resolve fevers.

The stimulating effects of Garlic are also felt in the digestive system, where it increases the flow of digestive enzymes and bile, improving absorption and assimilation of foods. Garlic is therefore helpful in indigestion, wind, abdominal discomfort, a generally sluggish digestion and constipation. Its effects on the pancreas improves the production and flow of insulin, making it useful to balance blood sugar levels. Garlic's anti-microbial actions also reduce acute or chronic digestive infections including candida, typhoid and cholera. Taken on an empty stomach, Garlic clears intestinal parasites. The regular use of Garlic establishes a healthy and balanced gut flora, in candida and after the use of antibiotics, and antidotes toxins and poisons, e.g. from food poisoning.

The warming and stimulating qualities of Garlic can also be beneficial to the circulation, where it helps to balance blood pressure, increases the flow of blood and lowers cholesterol levels. Taken long term, Garlic helps to resolve thrombosis and checks the development of arteriosclerosis.

As a powerful anti-oxidant, Garlic protects against the effects of stress and pollution and slows the ageing process.

Nicholas Culpeper described Garlic as a 'remedy for all diseases and hurts', but at the same time warns that its heat is 'very vehement'. He advises: 'Let it be taken inwardly with great moderation.'

The external use treats athlete's foot and vaginal thrush.

Dosage: 3–5 cloves a day.
　　　　　Tincture: 0.5–2 ml.

Caution: Avoid medicinal dosages in pregnancy and while breast feeding.

Large quantities of Garlic should be avoided by people prone to feeling very hot and dry and those with a sensitive digestion.

Ginger

Zingiber officinale, Zingiberaceae

Part used: Rhizome.

Constituents: Volatile oils, mucilage, resin.

Actions: Carminative, antiseptic, circulatory stimulant, diaphoretic, expectorant, rubefacient.

Uses: Ginger root is highly aromatic with a bitter-sweet and pungent taste.

The immediate effect when drinking or eating Ginger is a warming sensation in the abdomen before it spreads to all parts of the body imparting a sense of well-being and energy. Dioscorides describes Ginger as a remedy that eases everything that tenses and darkens the face.

Ginger is therefore used as a warming circulatory stimulant when suffering from cold hands and feet, chilblains, fatigue due to cold as well as aches and pains associated with chilliness.

Ginger also makes an excellent warming remedy with antiseptic, diaphoretic and expectorant qualities against colds, flu, bronchitis, sinusitis. It is prescribed for abdominal discomfort and distension, wind, colic, nausea and vomiting where the anti-spasmodic and carminative actions come to the fore. Chewed fresh, Ginger relieves motion sickness and, taken with care and moderation, eases morning sickness.

The warming, stimulating and anti-spasmodic effects of Ginger are also beneficial in scanty periods associated with menstrual cramps due to poor pelvic circulation. Likewise, it can be used in impotence where associated with deficient circulation.

Taken regularly, Ginger improves immunity, strengthens the adrenal glands and increases energy.

The fresh root makes a versatile remedy. It can be chewed fresh or prepared as a decoction to be drunk as a tea or applied as a warming compress. The infused oil finds use as a massage oil to relieve muscular and joint aches, period pains, to improve the circulation and boost energy.

While Ginger is a potent remedy in its own right, it is also well known to enhance the actions of other remedies. A pinch of Ginger often rounds off a herbal mixture and assists all remedies to reach their full potential.

Dosage: Decoction: 1–5 g.
            Tincture: 0.5–2 ml.

Caution: Ayurvedic medicine notes that people suffering from hyperacidity or gastric ulcers should avoid Ginger.

Hawthorn

Crataegus oxyacanthoides, Rosaceae

Part used: Berries, flowering tops.

Constituents: Flavonoids, saponins, acids, tannins, vitamin C, calcium.

Actions: Heart tonic, anti-spasmodic, hypotensive, diuretic, vasodilator, relaxant.

Uses: Hawthorn has long been considered a protective and sacred plant. Almost all parts have been used in healing, although nowadays it is mostly the berries and the flowering tops that are used medicinally.

Hawthorn is a subtle, gentle, yet highly potent remedy for the heart and the circulation. It acts as a heart tonic and nourishes the heart muscle, which, over time, restores coronary circulation and heart function. Its gentle diuretic effects complement the direct actions on the heart by relieving water retention. Hawthorn is therefore ideal for all heart conditions, including angina, arrythmia, tachycardia, breathing difficulties, degenerative heart diseases and heart failure.

Taken long term, Hawthorn regulates the whole circulatory system, improving the blood supply to all areas of the body. In addition, it softens deposits and hardened blood vessels. This makes it a valuable remedy to correct high or low blood pressure, particularly when associated with artherosclerosis or arteriosclerosis.

Hawthorn also has a relaxing effect on the nervous system, addressing anxiety, stress and depression so often experienced with heart and circulatory problems. When these problems are associated with nervous system overactivity such as palpitations, anxiety or insomnia, I tend to use the berries as they impart a calming peaceful autumn energy. Should circulatory problems be associated with lethargy and depression I draw on the uplifting, yet soothing energy of the fresh flowers and leaves gently to stimulate the vital spirits.

On an emotional level, Hawthorn, like other members of the Rose family, opens the heart, heals disappointment and rejection and facilitates the expression of love, where difficult issues have turned into inward or outward anger.

Hawthorn is best taken in small dosages over a period of 2–3 months, but can safely be taken continuously if required.

Dosage: Infusion: 6–14 g.
           Decoction: 6–16 g.
           Tincture: 3–6 ml.

Horsechestnut

Aesculus hippocastanum, Hippocastanaceae

Part used: Seed.

Constituents: Saponins, flavonoids, tannins, coumarins.

Actions: Astringent, anti-coagulant, anti-inflammatory, vasodilator.

Uses: The seeds of the Horsechestnut tree have affinity with the venous circulation and integrity of blood vessels.

By toning and strengthening the capillaries and blood vessels and also thinning the blood, thus improving the movement of blood through the whole circulation, Horsechestnut noticeably removes venous congestion of the abdomen and lower extremities. These can manifest as heavy, aching legs with cramps, especially at night, dull abdominal aches with constipation and bloating, haemorrhoids, varicose veins, varicose ulcers and thrombophlebitis. Likewise, heavy menstrual bleeding and dragging period pains as well as prostate enlargement can be an indication of pelvic congestion and may respond to treatment with Horsechestnut.

The astringency of the seed benefits not only the blood vessels, but also the mucous membranes of the digestive, respiratory and reproductive systems reducing diarrhoea, bronchitis, heavy menstrual bleeding and post-partum haemorrhage.

External application of Horsechestnut in the form of compresses, lotions, cream. complement the internal use in haemorrhoids, varicose veins and skin eruptions.

Dosage: Decoction: 3–6 g.
Tincture: 0.2–1 ml.

Cautions: Best used in conjunction with other remedies. Avoid before surgery or with bleeding disorders.

Horsetail

Equisetum arvense, Equisetaceae

Part used: Aerial.

Constituents: Salicylic acid, saponins, flavonoids, alkaloids, bitters, calcium, trace elements.

Actions: Astringent, diuretic, nutritive, vulnerary.

Uses: Horsetail is an excellent cooling astringent for both acute and chronic conditions of the genito-urinary, respiratory and digestive system.

The plant's astringency effectively reduces internal and external haemorrhages such as nosebleeds, passing of blood in the urine or stools, due to acute cystitis, prostatitis or diarrhoea, heavy menstrual bleeding with fibroids and endometriosis, menopausal fluctuations, miscarriage or still birth. Horsetail stops discharges from wounds, profuse sweating and excessive mucus in the respiratory or reproductive systems.

Horsetail contains significant amounts of calcium and silica which makes it an important nourishing plant with tonic and restorative properties. It is used in mineral deficiencies to revitalize the blood, including broken nails, split hair, osteoporosis and anaemia and to build bone and strengthen the skin, lung and kidney tissues.

While Horsetail acts as a mild diuretic useful for arthritic and skin complaints, its astringency and toning action also makes it effective in urinary incontinence and benign prostate enlargement.

Dosage: Decoction: 6–12 g.
          Tincture: 1–4 ml.

Caution: Horsetail is best used long-term with other herbs as it may cause urinary irritation if taken on its own for more than a few weeks.

Hydrangea

Hydrangea arborescens, Saxifragaceae

Part used: Root.

Constituents: Glycosides, alkaloids, saponins, resins, volatile oils, trace elements.

Actions: Diuretic.

Uses: The root of this evergreen shrub, well known for its cultivated garden variety, has long been praised as a herb for the urinary system.

Hydrangea can be used in acute bladder and urethra irritation with antiseptic and demulcent effects. It is specific for the treatment of prostatitis and enlargement of the prostate. When taken long term it is used to soften and eliminate urinary stones and gravel, especially when associated with infections.

In chronic toxic conditions, such as rheumatoid arthritis, gout and eczema the diuretic effect has a cleansing action on the whole body.

Dosage: Decoction: 8–14 g.
           Tincture: 2–4 ml.

Ladies' Mantle

Alchemilla vulgaris, Rosaceae

Part used: Aerial.

Constituents: Tannins, glycosides, saponins, bitters, salicylic acid.

Actions: Astringent, diuretic, emmenagogue, anti-inflammatory, vulnerary.

Uses: Ladies' Mantle is the herb of choice for conditions affecting women's reproductive health.

As a uterine tonic and emmenagogue it stimulates and balances the flow of periods, helps to reduce period pains and regulates irregular cycles. Due to the gradual increase in progesterone production, Ladies' Mantle harmonizes menstruation, pre-menstrual symptoms and the menopause. The combination of bitters and tannins strengthens and heals uterine tissue. It can be used in the treatment of heavy periods due to fibroids or around the menopause, for vaginal discharge with or without uterine infection and to heal any physical trauma suffered in the area. Ladies Mantle is effective in preparing for conception, especially when associated with low progesterone. It will help to support labour where it can be used to strengthen and stimulate contractions. After childbirth, it reduces heavy blood loss, heals where necessary and helps the womb to regain its natural size and prevent prolapse. After breast feeding it helps the breasts to regain tone and elasticity.

Used externally, Ladies' Mantle lotion acts as a wound healer in episiotomies, skin rashes and insect stings as well as eye and mouth inflammations. As a douche it staunches vaginal discharges.

While Ladies' Mantle is an excellent uterine tonic, it is also an alchemical plant that integrates and transforms female energies, giving women perspective and focus. I especially use it for women who need support to integrate their femaleness, to strengthen their sense of self and affirm their sexuality and creativity in order to ultimately embrace wider visions and possibilities for themselves.

Dosage: Infusion: 8–12 g.
          Tincture: 2–5 ml.

Caution: Avoid during pregnancy.

Lavender

Lavandula officinalis, Labiatae

Part used: Flowers.

Constituents: Volatile oils, tannins.

Actions: Carminative, anti-spasmodic, anti-depressant, anti-microbial, antiseptic, rubefacient.

Uses: Loved especially for its delightful fragrance, Lavender has been one of the most widely used medicinal herbs throughout the ages.

Lavender can be described as a deeply sympathetic and compassionate plant that addresses both acute and chronic conditions which require its harmonizing and balancing energy.

The flowers are well known for their actions on the nervous system, which, depending on need, can be either stimulating or relaxing.

In complaints associated with overactivity of the nervous system, such as agitation, anxiety, insomnia, high blood pressure, palpitations, irritability, migraines, Lavender tea will calm the spirits, reduce tension and promote rest and relaxation. Lavender is excellent to ease the effects of acute physical and emotional shock and trauma. Lack of vitality, nervous exhaustion and depression will draw on the warming and stimulating action of Lavender which improve the circulation, lift the spirits and increase physical and emotional energy.

Lavender relaxes the digestion and eases spasms and colic associated with tension and anxiety, but will also gently promote the flow of digestive juices, thereby improving sluggish bowel function.

The antiseptic volatile oils make Lavender a potent remedy for infections and inflammations of the skin, digestive and urinary system, including diarrhoea, cystitis, acne, eczema and parasites of the intestines and the skin. Applied externally, Lavender calms itchy skin, disinfects wounds and promotes healing. It soothes the pain of sprains and muscle aches.

Together with the antiseptic action of the volatile oils, the decongesting and expectorant action make Lavender a useful remedy for inflammations and infections of the respiratory system, especially where associated with tension and agitation. These include bronchitis, colds, flu and ear infections as well as coughs and asthma.

Lavender's capacity to alleviate pain makes it a comforting plant in chronic painful conditions such as arthritis and neuralgias as well as in relieving menstrual cramps, labour pains and headaches.

Dosage: Infusion: 8–12 g.
Tincture: 2–4 ml.

Caution: Avoid large quantities during pregnancy.

Lemon Balm

Melissa officinalis, Labiatae

Part used: Aerial.

Constituents: Volatile oils, bitters, tannins, acids, minerals.

Actions: Carminative, anti-spasmodic, anti-depressant, diaphoretic, hypotensive, anti-viral, anti-bacterial.

Uses: Lemon Balm was known as a cordial herb in the past, a remedy that affects the heart, but also lifts the spirits and balances the temperaments. Hildegard von Bingen praised its warmth that touches the spleen and delights the heart. Nicholas Culpeper writes that it strengthens nature much in all its actions. Research has shown that Lemon Balm influences the limbic system, that part of the brain concerned with emotions and the functions of the autonomic nervous system.

As a relaxing herb, Lemon Balm eases tension and irritability, including extreme anxiety, fear and phobias. When taken at night, it aids restful sleep. But it also lifts depression, mental and physical fatigue and calms long-term stresses, indicating its restoring and balancing effects on the nervous system. These effects are also noticeable in other parts of the body.

In the circulatory and respiratory system, the relaxing and restorative qualities ease complaints associated with hyperactivity, such as palpitations, high blood pressure, irregular heartbeat and breathing, wheezing, asthma and nervous coughs, tinnitus and headaches. It also helps to relax muscle spasm in the urinary system and eases menstrual cramps. Taken pre-menstrually or during the menopause, Lemon Balm can relieve associated irritability, mood swings and depression.

The volatile oils and bitters of the plant make it an important digestive remedy, relaxing spasms, indigestion and flatulence while gently stimulating liver and gall-bladder function and overall improving digestion.

Drunk as a hot infusion, Lemon Balm causes sweating and has cleansing effects in fevers and infections, including childhood infectious diseases, with specific anti-viral action against the herpes virus. Internal use can be complemented by external applications. Used externally, Lemon Balm also eases swellings, bruises, eye inflammations and insect stings.

Lemon Balm's overall qualities provide gentle warmth and nourishment. I use the herb for those caring for others who have become exhausted, depleted and disheartened. Lemon Balm will not only replenish their vitality and support their nervous system, but also warm and nourish the heart and help to rebuild a positive sense of self and identity. Women in the last few weeks of pregnancy enjoy Lemon Balm as it helps them to prepare emotionally and physically for the coming changes and challenges.

Dosage: Infusion: 8–16 g.
          Tincture: 2–5 ml.

Limeflower

Tilia europea, Tiliaceae

Part used: Flowers.

Constituents: Volatile oils, saponins, flavonoids, tannins, vitamin C.

Actions: Anti-spasmodic, diaphoretic, diuretic, sedative, hypotensive, anti-coagulant.

Uses: Limeflowers make a beautifully light and relaxing tea to relieve tension and anxiety and to aid restful sleep.

The sedative effects of Limeflower ease irritability, palpitations, agitation and tension headaches, as much as menstrual cramps, muscular spasms and tightness in neck and shoulders. In the treatment for addictions, Limeflower can be used to ease withdrawal symptoms although medication should only gradually be reduced.

Limeflower is also known for its beneficial effects on the circulation. The action of the flavonoids thin the blood and improve integrity of the blood vessels. These actions, together with the plant's relaxing and diuretic effects, make it a valuable remedy in arteriosclerosis, angina pectoris and to lower high blood pressure, especially when associated with stress and tension. Limeflower is especially helpful for people who have cut themselves off from their emotions and connections to others as it helps to release blocked emotional energy by warming and opening the heart and circulation.

Taken as hot infusion, Limeflower increases surface circulation and causes sweating. It has long been appreciated as a fever remedy and is excellent when drunk at the onset of respiratory infections such as colds, flu and sore throats, where it may also be used as a gargle.

Applied externally, the strong infusion will soothe burns and sore eyes and arrest bleeding and discharge from boils and abscesses.

Dosage: Infusion: 6–14 g.
              Tincture: 2–4 ml.

Liquorice

Glycyrrhiza glabra, Leguminosae

Part used: Root.

Constituents: Glycyrrhizin (terpene), saponins, flavonoids, oestrogenic substances, coumarin, bitters, volatile oils, tannins, starch (20%).

Actions: Demulcent, expectorant, anti-inflammatory, mild laxative, diuretic, adrenal tonic.

Uses: Liquorice root is much valued for healing dry inflammatory conditions of the digestive, respiratory and urinary systems. These uses can easily be deduced from the sweet taste of the root.

Through lowering stomach acids, Liquorice eases hyperacidity and heartburn and finds much use in the healing of gastric and peptic ulcers. It is said to have a protecting and detoxifying action on the liver and can be used in liver congestion, including hepatitis. It is mildly laxative.

In the respiratory system, Liquorice has similarly soothing and healing effects. It is widely used as a syrup in coughs, including whooping cough and bronchial infections. In addition, it lowers fevers and reduces allegic reactions in the respiratory system, such as asthma, allergic rhinitis and hayfever.

The demulcent and soothing qualities of the root are also noticeable in the urinary system where it eases the characteristic symptoms of irritation in cystitis and urethritis.

Due to compounds similar to those produced by the adrenal cortex, Liquorice can be used instead of steroid drugs in auto-immune disorders, and reduces the impact of their long term use. Imbalances due to oestrogen deficiencies, e.g. during the menopause, can be harmonized. Overall, it strengthens and tones the adrenal glands, increasing not only our ability to resist stress and exhaustion, but also enhancing and regulating immunity.

According to Nicholas Culpeper, Liquorice is 'the nearest to our temper' indicating its gentle, sweet yet deeply nourishing qualities.

Dosage: Decoction: 4–14 g.

Tincture: 1–4 ml.

Caution: Avoid with adrenal hyperfunction, in cardiovascular conditions and during pregnancy.

Marigold

Calendula officinalis, Compositae

Part used: Flower.

Constituents: Saponins, flavonoids, bitters, mucilage, resin, volatile oil.

Actions: Antiseptic, anti-fungal, anti-bacterial, anti-viral, astringent, bitter, diaphoretic, diuretic, emmenagogue, vulnerary, alterative, oestrogenic.

Uses: Marigold is a deep-acting anti-microbial herb and immune stimulant for use in both acute and chronic infections. It has been shown to be effective in acute herpes attacks, respiratory infections such as flu, colds and childhood infectious diseases, including mumps, chickenpox, measles, and in infections and inflammations in the bowels, such as gastritis and enteritis. Marigold is specific for both acute and chronic fungal infections such as vaginal thrush, athlete's foot and candidiasis (generalized fungus infection).

Drunk as a hot infusion, Marigold is diaphoretic and helps to sweat out toxins. A powerful blood and lymph cleanser, it can be used to clear chronic skin conditions and relieve lymphatic congestion.

Marigold has particular affinity for the female reproductive system. It effectively addresses infections and inflammations such as cervicitis, cervical erosion and pelvic inflammatory disease and heals wounds due to gynaecological surgery or difficult childbirth.

The oestrogenic properties and stimulant action on the uterus make Marigold an important remedy to regulate menstruation, ease painful periods when associated with pelvic congestion and check the heavy bleeding of fibroids, endometriosis and during the menopause. These actions are supported by the bitter properties stimulating the digestion and promoting better liver function which is needed to break down hormones effectively. In the treatment of pre-menstrual symptoms and menopausal fluctuations, Marigold helps to relieve irritability, water retention, tender swollen breasts and sluggish bowels.

Marigold flowers also have astringent properties which, due to the saponins and flavonoids, tone and restore venous and capillary circulation. Thus, Marigold heals varicose veins and haemorrhoids and eases heavy aching legs and cramps.

Marigold's potent wound-healing capacities can be seen in both internal and external use. In the digestive tract, Marigold heals gastric and peptic ulcers and any irritation of the mucous membranes of the mouth and oesophagus. Externally Marigold swiftly staunches bleeding, prevents infections, promotes tissue repair and reduces swelling and scar formations.

Many external preparations of Marigold are useful and range from the application of the fresh, bruised flowers to compresses, mouthwashes and creams.

Emotionally, Marigold is helpful for those in need of protection. Associated with the solar plexus, Marigold enables us to be more discriminating when tempted to take on the emotional burdens of others.

Dosage: Infusion: 8–14 g.
             Tincture: 2–4 ml.

Caution: Avoid internal use during pregnancy.

Marshmallow

Althaea officinalis, Malvaceae

Part used: Root, leaves.

Constituents: *Roots*: mucilage (up to 35%), pectin, tannins, calcium, trace elements; *Leaf*: mucilage, volatile oils.

Actions: Demulcent, expectorant, diuretic, emollient.

Uses: The root has a starchy, sweet taste indicating its profusion of mucilage with attendant soothing, cooling and moisturizing actions. It is an important remedy for any hot, dry conditions of the mucous membranes and the skin.

In the digestive system, Marshmallow relieves hyperacidity, gastritis and ulcers and supports the healing of irritated and inflamed stomach lining. It soothes the bowels in acute diarrhoea, such as gastro-enteritis and dysentery, and harmonizes peristalsis in colitis with alternating constipation and diarrhoea.

As a soothing expectorant, Marshmallow will ease dry, irritating and unproductive coughs, such as tickly coughs, whooping cough, pleurisy, bronchitis and pneumonia and moisturize dry, sore mouth and throat. A syrup is particularly effective in respiratory conditions.

In the urinary system, Marshmallow acts as a soothing diuretic and is especially effective in infections characterized by burning, painful and frequent urination. It is therefore commonly used in cystitis, urethritis and nephritis and has also been used to help flush out urinary gravel.

Marshmallow is also said to promote lactation, and Dioscorides describes the root as a remedy to ease the passage of the afterbirth and staunch post-natal discharges.

Externally, Marshmallow makes an excellent gargle for sore throats and mouth; a poultice will cool skin rashes and insect bites and draw out splinters, boils and abscesses. In the past Marshmallow ointment was commonly used to ease stiff joints and muscles and relieve aches, sprains and bruising.

Both the root and the leaves can be used, although generally the root is more mucilaginous.

Dosage: *Leaf*: Infusion: 8–14 g.
          Root: Decoction: 6–16 g.
          Tincture: 2–4 ml.

Meadowsweet

Filipendula ulmaria, Rosaceae

Part used: Aerial.

Constituents: Salicylic glycosides, salicylic acids, flavonoids, tannins, volatile oils, mucilage, iron, sulphur, calcium, silica, vitamin C.

Actions: Anti-rheumatic, anti-inflammatory, astringent, diaphoretic, diuretic, anacid, analgesic.

Uses: Meadowsweet has a long history as an analgesic in inflammatory conditions and fever. On crushing, it releases the typical smell of salicylic aldehydes which the body converts to salicylic acid. This was first prepared in pure form in 1836 and subsequently synthesized as Aspirin.

Herbally, Meadowsweet is used in arthritic, rheumatic and gouty joint pains with redness, heat and swelling general aches and pains, childhood infections as well as fevers. The diuretic and diaphoretic actions at the same time help to eliminate toxic wastes from the body. Meadowsweet is rich in vitamin C, magnesium, silica and calcium, which explains its ability to speed the healing of all connective tissues and mucous membranes as well as wounds, cuts and skin irritations when applied externally. Meadowsweet also softens deposits such as kidney and bladder stones and hardened arteries.

The combination of tannins and mucilage in the plant make it an invaluable antacid and anti-inflammatory remedy. It can be used for a wide range of digestive complaints associated with hyperacidity and inflammation such as diarrhoea, heartburn, gastritis, peptic ulcers and irritable bowel as well as cystitis and urethritis.

It is a gentle, yet deep-acting remedy which is generally well-tolerated by sensitive people, children and the elderly.

Dosage: Infusion: 6–16 g.
Tincture: 2–5 ml.

Caution: Meadowsweet affects the blood-clotting rate and should be avoided in blood-clotting diseases and when taking anti-coagulants.

Mullein

Verbascum thapsus, Scrophulariaceae

Part used: Leaves, flowers.

Constituents: Mucilage, volatile oils, resin, saponins, flavonoids, tannins, trace elements.

Actions: Expectorant, demulcent, diuretic, anti-spasmodic, mild astringent, vulnerary.

Uses: Mullein is an excellent all-round respiratory herb with uses ranging from sore throats to pain in the chest. It is soothing in dry irritating coughs, laryngitis and sore throats, where Hildegard von Bingen recommends it in combination with Fennel. In chronic respiratory conditions such as asthma and bronchitis the saponins help to loosen phlegm and stimulate expectoration. A syrup is the preferred preparation for the respiratory system.

Like other herbs with a high mucilage content, Mullein infusion eases digestive irritation such as diarrhoea. As a soothing diuretic, Mullein will relieve the burning and frequency of urination in acute cystitis and urethritis and gently remove toxins via the kidneys in arthritis and rheumatism and swollen lymph glands. Should the infusion be prepared with the flowers, the tea needs to be thoroughly strained so that the fine hairs do not irritate the mucous membranes.

The flowers are frequently applied externally as a poultice or a cream to soften boils and draw pus, splinters and other toxins in sores and skin infections.

Exposing the blossoms in a tightly closed bottle to the heat of the sun will, after a few days, extract a mucilaginous, watery essence which, once strained, is very effective in earaches, middle ear infection, hearing loss and loss of balance. Alternatively, an infused oil can be prepared for the same purpose.

Dosage: Infusion: 6–14 g.
         Tincture: 2–4 ml.

Nettle

Urtica dioica, Urticacea

Part used: Aerial.

Constituents: Formic acid, chlorophyll, tannins, mucilage, histamine, serotonin, vitamins B, C, carotenes, iron, magnesium, potassium, trace elements.

Actions: astringent, diuretic, nutritive, tonic.

Uses: The excellent nourishing and restoring effects of Nettle leaves largely depend on its high content of vitamins and trace elements, proteins, carotene and chlorophyll. It strengthens the blood, renews connective tissue, promotes healthy intestinal flora, activates enzymes and improves liver and pancreatic functions. Nettle is therefore used where there is any loss of energy and vitality, such as fatigue, anaemia, liver imbalances and pancreatitis.

Partly due to the plant's high chlorophyll content, it also reduces fungal and yeast proliferation in the gut and, when used externally, bacterial overgrowth of wounds.

While immensely nourishing, Nettle is at the same time also profoundly cleansing and has long been valued as an important spring tonic. Taken fresh throughout March, the warming and drying quality of Nettle will remove accumulated winter phlegm. Culpepper recommends Nettle with honey to stimulate expectoration and to relieve coughing in bronchitis and other respiratory infections. Nettle generally removes toxic waste from the body and softens and dissolves hard deposits such as urinary gravel and kidney and gall stones. Nettle improves arthritic, gouty and rheumatic conditions with high uric acid accumulation and clears chronic skin problems such as psoriasis, eczema and dandruff. As a diuretic Nettle is helpful wherever water retention or difficult urination is present.

The astringency is effective in diarrhoea, urinary infections and infections of the mouth and throat. It reduces heavy menstrual bleeding and when taken long term in conjunction with other herbs will restore hormonal balance. Nettle root, however, is used traditionally to reduce benign enlargement of the prostate although I have found that the fresh herb is also effective.

Externally, washes and compresses are used in arthritic conditions to improve local circulation and provide pain relief. For dry scalp, lacklustre and falling hair, a vinegar decoction with Nettle and Rosemary is highly recommended. Made into a cream or ointment, Nettle is particularly suitable for skin conditions.

Dosage: Infusion: 10–20 g.
Tincture: 4–6 ml.

Oats

Avena sativa, Graminaceae

Part used: Whole plant.

Constituents: Starch, alkaloids, proteins, flavonoids, saponins, vitamins B1 and 2, D, E, P, carotene, minerals, trace elements calcium, silica, magnesium, iron.

Actions: demulcent, nervine tonic, anti-depressant, vulnerary, nutritive.

Uses: Oats are food and medicine in one, being nourishing and restoring at the same time. They are rich in vitamins and minerals and have a warm nature with a sweet and slightly bitter taste.

Eaten regularly, Oats provide nourishment in chronic fatigue, exhaustion, anaemia, convalescence and general debility. They strengthen the immune system, support the nervous system and restore hormonal balance. Taken long term, Oats protect against heart attack as they remove cholesterol from the digestion and the arteries. Being rich in silica, calcium and magnesium, Oats help to renew and strengthen muscles, bones, cartilage and teeth during rapid development in childhood and adolescence as well as in arthritis and osteoporosis.

Oats are easily digested and soothing to mucous membranes. They are therefore helpful to ease irritated digestion due to increased acidity. Similarly, Oats can be used effectively in bladder irritation or with dry irritating coughs.

Prepared as decoction or tincture, Oats restore the nervous system whereby their relaxing and grounding, yet toning qualities come to the fore. Oats can be used long term to treat anxiety, depression, nervous and emotional exhaustion, sleep disorders, lack of concentration, memory loss and headaches due to overstimulation. Oats are often used to support people during withdrawal from addictive substances.

Applied externally, Oats make a soothing addition to a bath for irritating skin conditions such as eczema. A hot compress can be used for painful arthritic joints, to draw toxins from boils and abscesses and to ease itchy inflamed skin.

Dosage: As food.
Decoction: 10–20 g.
Tincture: 2–4 ml.

Caution: People with gluten intolerance should avoid all Oat preparations.

Peppermint

Mentha piperita, Labiatae

Part used: Aerial.

Constituents: Volatile oils, tannins, flavonoids, bitters, resin.

Actions: carminative, anti-spasmodic, anti-emetic, diaphoretic, bitter, antiseptic, astringent, nervine, decongestant.

Uses: Dioscorides describes Mint as warming, binding and drying and already in those times Mint was particularly recommended for the digestion.

Peppermint is a reliable digestive aid when nausea, travel sickness, indigestion or acute vomiting require immediate attention. A warm infusion sipped slowly will offer much relief. Relaxing smooth muscles, Peppermint eases complaints associated with discomfort due to muscular spasms in the digestive system such as colic, IBS, flatulence, diarrhoea, constipation and colitis. The tannins help to protect the mucous membranes against infection and inflammation, such as parasites, cholera, enteritis, herpes simplex and zoster. In addition, as a stimulant to the liver and pancreas, Peppermint improves liver and gall bladder congestion manifesting in sluggish digestion and bowel function, hepatitis, gall stones and migraines associated with digestive complaints.

Peppermint is both a warming and cooling herb depending on the preparation and the condition it is used for. Drunk as a hot infusion, Peppermint is a valuable fever remedy increasing sweating, the release of toxins and ultimately cooling to the body temperature.

The volatile oils are strongly anti-viral and anti-bacterial. An infusion wards off colds and flu, reduces mucus production and relieves catarrh. Peppermint makes a useful gargle for sore throats and inhalations for sinusitis, bronchitis and ear infections.

In smaller but frequent dosage, the infusion tends to be stimulating and balancing to the circulation, especially when associated with headaches, heat and dizziness. Peppermint makes a pleasant general tonic improving loss of concentration, lack of vitality and debility.

Compresses, being cooling and numbing, ease rheumatic and neuralgic pain, sciatica, toothache and itching and irritated skin inflammations.

Dosage: Infusion: 3–7 g.
            Tincture: 1–3 ml.

Caution: Large dosages may cause epileptic seizures.

Raspberry

Rubus idaeus, Rosaceae

Part used: Leaf.

Constituents: Tannins, alkaloids, acids, vitamins C, A, calcium, iron, trace elements.

Actions: Astringent, anti-spasmodic, uterine tonic, parturient.

Uses: Raspberry is a very widely used and effective uterine tonic. It tones the muscles of the pelvic region in general and specifically the muscles of the uterus, helps to build as well as restore uterine tissue and harmonizes uterine functions.

Much of the strengthening and balancing qualities ascribed to Raspberry are due to the effects of the alkaloids as well as the profound nourishment provided by the vitamins and minerals, which are easily assimilated.

Taken regularly, Raspberry harmonizes uterine functions, especially when associated with painful, scanty periods or heavy bleeding whereby the astringency reduces blood loss. Being gentle and gradually balancing, Raspberry is suitable for young women, should their cycle need subtle support in finding its own rhythm.

As part of pre-conception care, Raspberry is an excellent herb to increase fertility in both women and men. As Raspberry tones and strengthens the uterine muscles, it can help to prevent miscarriges due to an overrelaxed or atonic uterus.

By releasing tension in the digestive system and increasing astringency, Raspberry leaves are helpful to relieve diarrhoea, particularly in children, and also heartburn and indigestion. In pregnancy, the infusion can ease morning sickness.

By toning the muscles needed during pregnancy and labour, Raspberry encourages the contracting uterus to work more effectively, making the birth easier while also reducing recovery time. During pregnancy and after delivery, the leaves are best taken as a warm infusion. In the first two trimesters, one cup per day is sufficient, although this may be increased to counter morning sickness and a threatened miscarriage. During the last two to three months enjoy two to three cups per day. Should you be feeling tense and anxious before birth, mix Raspberry with Lemon Balm or Chamomile in order to relax and avoid holding negative emotional tension in the pelvis as this may interfere with labour.

Raspberry syrup of the fruits is prepared on the Continent to reduce inflammations and irritations in the mouth, throat, larynx and the lungs, including coughs and bronchitis. Children particularly enjoy the syrup.

Dosage: Infusion: 8–14 g.
Tincture: 2–4 ml.

Red Clover

Trifolium pratense, Leguminoscue

Part used: Flowers.

Constituents: acids, volatile oils, glycosides, coumarins, flavonoids, tannins, bitters, chlorophyll, vitamin C, minerals.

Actions: Alterative, anti-spasmodic, expectorant.

Uses: Red Clover flowers are a deep-acting alterative and blood cleanser for chronic conditions of toxicity with relaxing and anti-spasmodic properties.

It is helpful for long-standing eczema, psoriasis and other chronic skin complaints as well as malignant and benign tumours of the skin, breast and ovaries where the profound cleansing of the lymphatic system, together with the increased elimination of waste through the urinary system leads to normalization of tissue growth. It is of similar benefit in rheumatic and arthritic conditions.

With its affinity for the female reproductive system and an oestrogenic action, Red Clover can also be used to address chronic gynaecological conditions such as pelvic inflammatory disease, endometriosis and fibroids. Pre-menstrual symptoms associated with skin conditions such as acne benefit from the cleansing and balancing effects of Red Clover.

In the respiratory system the relaxant and anti-spasmodic properties of Red Clover combine with a soothing expectorant action. It eases dry irritating coughs, dry mouth and throat and coughs with severe bronchial spasms as seen in asthma, whooping cough and measles. A syrup would be the most suitable preparation, while a gargle will ease sore throats and laryngitis.

Red Clover likewise eases urinary irritation and reduces inflammation in cystitis, urethritis and other urinary and vaginal infections.

Externally, an infusion can be used as a wash for sore nipples, eye infections, insect stings, wounds and slow healing sores and skin ulcers.

Dosage: Infusion: 10–16 g.
Tincture: 2–4 ml.

Ribwort

Plantago lanceolata, Plantagincaeae

Part used: Leaf.

Constituents: Glycosides, tannins, mucilage, bitters, volatile oils, vitamins A, C, K, minerals, trace elements.

Actions: Demulcent, expectorant, astringent, diuretic.

Uses: Throughout history, Ribwort has been a respected wound healer. Nicholas Culpepper writes: 'The Plantains are singularly good wound herbs, to heal fresh or old wounds and sores, either inward or outward.' Dioscorides in addition, recommends fresh Ribwort juice for bites and stings and Hildegard von Bingen suggests compresses to heal broken bones.

Traditionally, Ribwort has been used for a wide range of acute conditions characterized by swelling, heat and irritation with or without discharge. Externally, the leaves staunch bleeding, ease pain, reduce infections and are used for wounds, skin and mouth ulcers, insect bites, burns and rashes. A poultice or the infusion of the fresh leaf used as a wash is most effective.

Taken internally, Ribwort is a renowned healer for the respiratory system where a syrup is the preferred preparation. It is used for the treatment of dry, tickly coughs with little phlegm where its effect is cooling and soothing while facilitating productive expectoration. It is equally effective in acute coughs with thick, yellow mucus whereby Ribwort inhibits excessive mucus production. In addition, it addresses infections of the upper respiratory system, including middle ear infections, sinusitis and acute rhinitis and hay fever.

Taken regularly, Ribwort, with its high silica content, strengthens the lungs and eases wheezing and asthma and reduces the damaging effects of poor air quality and smoking.

Acute digestive, urinary and uterine infections such as diarrhoea, dysentery, vaginal discharges and pelvic inflammation also benefit from the healing qualities of Ribwort.

For all these conditions, Ribwort is best used fresh. Alternatively use as a tincture prepared with fresh leaves, as on crushing the leaves form strong anti-bacterial qualities.

Dosage: Infusion: 8–16 g.
              Tincture: 2–4 ml.

Rosemary

Rosemarinus officinalis, Labiatae

Part used: Leaf.

Constituents: Volatile oils, saponins, flavonoids, tannins, resin, bitters, minerals.

Actions: Carminative, anti-spasmodic, antiseptic, bitter, astringent, circulatory stimulant, anti-depressant, relaxant, diuretic.

Uses: Rosemary's medicinal use centres on its overall stimulating and warming qualities. The stimulating effect on the heart and circulation relieves low blood pressure, cold extremities and dizziness as well as exhaustion and lack of vitality as the heart more effectively circulates the blood to all parts of the body. In doing so, Rosemary also relieves tightness of the chest with shortness of breath, palpitations, and wheezing. Overall the effect is restoring to circulatory deficiencies. Poor pelvic circulation also benefits from the regular use of Rosemary. Warming and stimulating, the flow of blood improves, easing painful, scanty periods, low fertility and increasing sexual energy in both women and men.

Drunk as a hot infusion, Rosemary promotes sweating, useful during the onset of colds, coughs and flu and eases acute aches and pains, aids expectoration in both acute and chronic coughs and clears congested sinuses and headaches.

The bitter taste of the plant stimulates the digestion. Together with the relaxant properties, it improves indigestion, nausea, wind, constipation, liver congestion and gall bladder irritation. By aiding liver function, Rosemary will help to remove toxins from the body which may account for its frequent use in all conditions associated with liverishness, from hangovers to irritability to loss of appetite.

Used externally, the addition of a strong infusion to a bath is an excellent energy booster. The diluted essential oil makes an invigorating massage oil and relieves menstrual cramps and aching muscles and joints, where associated with chills. Rubbed into the scalp, it is a good hair and scalp tonic.

Being warming by bringing blood to the surface of the skin, Rosemary also helps to speed wound healing and checks infections in cuts, grazes, sores, bruises and is effective in treating lice and scabies.

Emotionally, Rosemary is helpful for those who need to open their heart in order to balance their emotions and perceive the flow of inner harmony.

Dosage: Infusion: 6–12 g.
               Tincture: 2–4-ml.

Caution: Rosemary is best avoided long term with hypertension and if prone to excessive heat.

Sage

Salvia officinalis, Labiatae

Part used: Leaf.

Constituents: Volatile oils, saponins, flavonoids, bitters, oestrogenic substances, vitamins A, C, riboflavin, niacin, minerals (especially calcium, magnesium, iron, zinc).

Action: Antiseptic, astringent, anti-spasmodic, bitter, oestrogenic, diaphoretic, nervine and adrenal tonic, emmenagogue.

Uses: Sage is a potent anti-microbial remedy reducing infection in both the respiratory and digestive systems. The hot infusion acts as a diaphoretic and helps to check fevers at the onset of colds and flu, especially when associated with sore throats. Its drying and astringent qualities make it useful in sinusitis, tonsillitis, bronchitis and catarrh and chronic infections of the mouth. It is a trusted remedy for lung TB and other infections associated with night sweats. In chronic conditions Sage eases a tight chest, reduces wheezing and facilitates expectoration of phlegm.

As a digestive remedy, Sage warms the system and relaxes spasms, stimulates appetite and improves liver and digestive function. It can be used for indigestion, loose stools, mucus colitis, wind, nausea, enteritis and intestinal worms.

The volatile oils found in Sage are known to affect particularly the pituitary and adrenal glands. This confirms the long-standing use of Sage as a women's tonic. Where there is weakness and deficiency of the endocrine functions Sage harmonizes sex hormones and overall enhances immunity. It regulates menstruation, improves fertility when accompanied by low oestrogen levels, scanty or absent periods or a slow and weak onset of flow. It eases menstrual spasms and reduces pre-menstrual symptoms of irritability and fatigue with lack of concentration or depression. Sage can also reduce the heavy bleeding so common during puberty and the menopause whereby, in the latter, it also will improve hot flushes, night sweats, irritability, exhaustion and depression. As Sage can be rather drying, care should be taken with prolonged use (over weeks and months), if there is a tendency to dry skin and vagina.

During difficult and prolonged child birth, Sage can improve weak contractions and help to expel the placenta. Because of this stimulating effect on the uterus, Sage is contra-indicated in pregnancy. It should also be avoided while breast feeding as it may reduce the milk supply. This same property, however, makes it excellent when ready to wean.

The tonic benefits of Sage on the adrenal glands and the nervous system restore balanced function in chronic conditions such as auto-immune disorders, chronic debility and nervous exhaustion from prolonged emotional and physical stress, fatigue, low blood pressure, poor concentration and lack of mental focus and depression. For long-term use in this context, it is best combined with a nervine tonic such as Vervain, Wood Betony, Skullcap or Oats.

Applied externally, Sage washes promote healing and are excellent for wounds, cuts, burns, skin inflammation, ulcers and mouth and gum diseases; a vaginal douche relieves discharge and infections such as thrush, vaginal bacteriosis and chlamydia.

I have found Sage an excellent remedy with particular affinity for people who need to clear emotional obstructions and stagnation in order to allow for the flow of creativity and a balanced integration of physical, emotional and spiritual energies.

Dosage: Infusion: 6–12 g.
           Tincture: 1–4 ml.

Caution: Contra-indicated in pregnancy and while breast feeding.

Skullcap

Scutellaria laterifolia, Labiatae

Part used: Aerial.

Constituents: Volatile oils, flavonoids, tannins, bitters, iron, silica.

Actions: Nervine tonic, anti-spasmodic, astringent, diuretic, relaxant.

Uses: Like other members of the Mint family, Skullcap has specific affinity for the nervous system. The volatile oils and nutritive components of the plant restore an overstimulated and irritated nervous system while at the same time inducing rest and relaxation. Skullcap deeply strengthens and supports in times of prolonged stress manifesting as tension, anxiety, agitation, headaches, sleeping problems and depression and exhaustion. As a herb with an overall relaxing quality, Skullcap also eases chest pains, palpitations, panic attacks, shortness of breath and high blood pressure when associated with stress and anxiety.

Its anti-spasmodic action is useful in conditions associated with overexcitement such as nervous ticks, twitching, jerking muscles and trembling as well as epilepsy.

The use of Skullcap has proved helpful in overcoming the varied symptoms associated with withdrawal from addictive substances.

In addition, Skullcap is a bitter diuretic and digestive remedy. It can be used to ease urinary irritation, arthritic pain aggravated by stress, indigestion and loss of appetite.

Dosage: Infusion: 8–14 g.
          Tincture: 2–4 ml.

St John's Wort

Hypericum perforatum, Hypericaceae

Part used: Aerial.

Constituents: Volatile oils, tannins, flavonoids, resin.

Actions: Anti-depressant, relaxant, anti-spasmodic, anti-inflammatory, analgesic, astringent, anti-microbial, vulnerary.

Uses: St John's Wort is probably best known for its uplifting action on the nervous system, whereby it enhances the effects of neurotransmitters and positively influences serotonin-melatonin concentrations in the brain.

It is widely used as a tonic remedy for conditions of the nervous system that are characterized by nervous tension, spasms, exhaustion, sleep disturbances, melancholy and depression. The restoring effects, noticable only after the prolonged use of two–three months, facilitate relaxation and gradually replenish and restore vital energies. Its uplifting quality, when gentle yet effective support in times of increased demands is needed, has led to the common popular use as a 'herbal anti-depressant'. As St John's Wort also sensitizes the body to ultra-violet light, it can be used effectively by those suffering from lack of sunlight during the winter months. For the same reason, however, excessive exposure to sunlight while taking St John's Wort may cause skin irritation in sensitive people.

In addition, St John's Wort is an excellent remedy to ease nerve pain due to injury, irritation and inflammation. For best results in treating neuralgias, sciatica, arthralgias and spinal pains, the internal use should be complemented with external applications in the form of an infused oil, compress or ointment.

As a relaxing remedy that eases tension and spasms, St John's Wort can also be used to relieve menstrual cramps, colic and irritation in the digestive system, tension headaches and urinary incontinence when associated with irritation, pain and nervous excitement.

Much neglected is St John's Wort's potent efficacy as a first aid remedy. In the treatment of acute burns, cuts and wounds with inflammation and pain, it excels as a topical remedy with anti-inflammatory and pain-relieving as well as anti-viral and anti-bacterial properties. It is also useful in sprains, haemorrhoids, varicose veins and slow-healing ulcers. Viral skin conditions such as herpes, shingles and children's infections and skin conditions also benefit from internal and external use. I frequently use it with great success in ear infections.

Dosage: Infusion: 8–14 g.
       Tincture: 2–4 ml.

Caution: May cause sensitivity to sun light discontinue if necessary; use with caution during pregnancy; if on prescribed medication, consult a qualified practitioner.

Thyme

Thymus vulgaris, Labiatae

Part used: Leaves and flowers.

Constituents: Volatile oils, bitters, tannins, flavonoids, saponins, resins.

Actions: Anti-microbial, anthelmintic, carminative, anti-spasmodic, astringent, expectorant, tonic.

Uses: Thyme is a potent anti-microbial remedy with drying and bitter qualities and a typical pungent aroma. It can be used wherever there is a bacterial, viral or fungal infection, although it is particularly suitable to the respiratory, digestive, urinary and reproductive systems.

Drunk freely as a hot infusion, Thyme induces sweating, reduces fevers and checks infections. It therefore is used at the onset of colds, flu, sinusitis, laryngitis etc. It checks respiratory catarrh and eases both dry irritating and full productive coughs. Even severe respiratory infections such as chronic bronchitis, asthma, croup and whooping cough benefit from the expectorant, antiseptic action of Thyme with its warming and drying qualities which open the chest, dilate bronchioles and relax respiratory muscles. Thyme syrup is the most effective preparation for respiratory complaints.

Together with the warming and drying qualities, the bitter action is helpful in nausea, indigestion and wind. Candida, intestinal parasites and infections leading to diarrhoea and fermentation in the bowels respond well to Thyme as it addresses a wide range of intestinal microbes.

It is also a potent remedy for urinary and uterine infections accompanied by vaginal discharges, delayed, scanty menstruation and retained placenta.

Taken long term, Thyme, similar to Sage and Rosemary, restores the nervous system and adrenal glands and enhances immunity. It therefore can be used with great effect in general exhaustion, lack of vitality and mental focus together with a tendency to low resistance, respiratory and digestive infections, poor breathing patterns or asthma.

Compresses, washes, lotions and ointments are useful to treat athlete's foot, infected wounds and skin irritations. Whole body baths are especially recommended in respiratory infections, with rheumatic and arthritic pains and general exhaustion. Steam inhalations relieve respiratory congestion due to infections.

Dosage: Infusion: 4–10 g.

Tincture: 2-4 ml.

Caution: Contra-indicated in pregnancy; use with care in thyroid conditions.

Vervain

Verbena officinalis, Labiatae

Part used: Aerial.

Constituents: Volatile oils, glycosides, bitters, tannins, mucilage.

Actions: Nervine tonic, relaxant, anti-spasmodic, bitter, diaphoretic, diuretic, galactagogue, emmenagogue.

Uses: Vervain is a subtle, adaptive tonic for the nervous system with a wide range of benefits essential in holistic practice. It can be used for a multitude of nervous disorders ranging from oversensitivity to anxiety, stress, tension, irritation, confusion, lack of concentration, headaches, depression, insomnia and nervous exhaustion. Taken long term, Vervain is excellent to restore balance and function in the nervous system, building strength and resilience and relaxing an overactive adrenal gland.

Vervain's relaxing effects combine well with its bitter components in the treatment of digestive complaints associated with nervous tension such as indigestion, wind, colicky pain, irritable bowels, as Vervain stimulates the digestion and liver and helps to regulate sluggish function. It is said also to be effective against parasites.

When taken as a tepid infusion, Vervain exhibits a noticeable diuretic effect. Hence, musculoskeletal conditions associated with pain such as arthritis and gout as well as kidney and urinary gravel and skin diseases, benefit from its cleansing action.

The herb's generally relaxing and anti-spasmodic effects also ease tension and spasms in other parts of the body. It eases asthma and tight chests, palpitations, increased blood pressure associated with stress, period pains and slow, sluggish onset of menstruation. As Vervain is stimulating to the uterus, it should not be used during pregnancy, but can promote slow or stalled labour. It is beneficial while breast feeding as it increases milk production.

Vervain is an excellent fever herb when drunk as a hot infusion. It increases sweating, promotes elimination of toxins and lowers the body temperature. Use at the onset of colds, flu, children's infections and with intermittent fevers. It speeds recovery and has been found useful during convalescence from infections, including post-viral syndrome. Likewise, use it freely as a prophylactic during times of digestive or respiratory epidemics as it stimulates and supports immunity.

As an astringent mouthwash, Vervain is used for inflamed, bleeding gums and mouth and tongue ulcers. A gargle offers relief in laryngitis, tonsillitis and with sore throats. A lotion can be used to heal cuts, wounds and ease insect bites.

Vervain is a deep-acting herb, particularly suited to people who are in need of integrating their intellectual concerns with their emotional and physical beings in order to harmonize their energies and experience balanced well-being. Due to its gentle nature and breadth of actions it is frequently used for children.

Dosage: Infusion: 6–16 g.
Tincture: 2–5 ml.

Caution: Avoid during pregnancy.

White Willow

Salix alba, Salicaceae

Part used: Bark.

Constituents: Glycosides, salicin, flavonoids, tannins, resin.

Actions: Anti-inflammatory, anti-pyretic, analgesic, antiseptic, astringent.

Uses: White Willow bark is an excellent antiseptic fever remedy which can be used for acute infections with raised temperature such as throat, mouth, eye infections, urinary and digestive infections. It is also an effective herb for chronic conditions such as arthritic and rheumatic joint inflammations where the presence of salicin converted to salicylic acid on oxidation in the body offers additional pain relief. Headaches and neuralgic pains respond well to White Willow bark as well. The mildly bitter and diuretic properties make it a useful herb in the holistic treatment of such conditions as it gently stimulates the appetite and digestion and facilitates the elimination of toxins. Its astringent properties help to check diarrhoea and general discharges as well as heavy menstrual bleeding, nosebleeds and bleeding wounds. A compress eases cuts and wounds and a gargle treats bleeding gums and mouth ulcers.

I find Willow useful for people who have high expectations of themselves and easily feel bitterness, anger and frustration due to impatience with themselves and others.

Dosage: Decoction: 7–10 g.
　　　　　Tincture: 2–4 ml.

Wood Betony

Stachys betonica, Labiatae

Part used: Aerial.

Constituents: Alkaloids, glycosides, tannins, bitters, volatile oils.

Actions: Nervine tonic, relaxant, bitter, astringent.

Uses: Ancient Greek physicians described Wood Betony as a soul nourisher, a relaxing nervine tonic.

Conditions such as chronic exhaustion, nervous tension, depression, headaches, migraines and sleep disturbances respond well to Wood Betony especially when associated with fearfulness and anxiety. Deeply relaxing to the nervous system, it deflects the influences of negative attitudes and allows the release of tension and spasms. This engenders a sense of profound physical, emotional and mental well-being. It helps children and adults alike to overcome the unsettling fear of failure and lack of confidence and to face the demands of changes, especially when growing up, with greater equanimity. Use for nightmares, exam stress and the emotional fluctuations of adolescence and the menopause.

High blood pressure, palpitations, dizziness and fainting when due to stress and anxiety will be eased as will be tightness in the chest area, wheezing, asthma and coughs. If menstruation is a time characterized by anxiety and tension, pre-menstrual irritation and irritability, painful cramps and slow, difficult periods, Wood Betony can be called on to induce harmony. Equally, slow, difficult child birth can be facilitated through the relaxing quality of Wood Betony.

The bitters in Wood Betony will help to stimulate the digestion and liver and relieve constipation while the diuretic properties will relieve scanty urination and water retention. This will be of benefit in sluggish liver conditions, nervous indigestion and poor appetite, but also in painful arthritic and rheumatic complaints and irritating skin rashes. The tannins make it an excellent astringent remedy for diarrhoea, heavy menstrual bleeding, vaginal discharges and mouth and throat infections. Used externally, Wood Betony speeds wound healing in sores, ulcers, varicose veins and haemorrhoids.

Wood Betony is especially useful for people of all ages who easily worry, and are fearful and anxious.

Dosage: Infusion: 8–12 g.
            Tincture: 2–4 ml.

Caution: Avoid in pregnancy.

Yarrow

Achillea millefolium, Compositae

Part used: Aerial.

Constituents: Volatile oils, alkaloids, tannins, resins, salicylic acid, flavonoids, saponins, vitamin C, minerals, potassium 48%.

Actions: Anti-inflammatory, diaphoretic, anti-spasmodic, antiseptic, diuretic, carminative, bitter astringent, emmenagogue, vulnerary.

Uses: During the early Middle Ages, Yarrow was called 'Eyebrows of Venus' indicating with other plants dedicated to Venus, its use for healing women's complaints. Modern pharmacology confirms Yarrow as a versatile gynaecological remedy exerting hormonal influences and regulating menstruation from puberty through to the menopause. In addition, Yarrow stimulates and tones venous circulation, removing pelvic congestion and harmonizing uterine blood flow. Yarrow is therefore used to improve amenorrhoea and scanty periods by toning and warming the pelvic organs as well as checking heavy menstrual bleeding, whereby the tannins contribute an astringent action. A range of volatile oils provide a relaxing quality much needed to ease tension, discomfort and spasms of menstrual cramps and relieve physical and emotional symptoms occurring pre-menstrually.

The decongesting, toning and relaxing qualities are also helpful to relieve conditions manifesting in the circulation in general such as varicose veins, haemorrhoids, heavy, painful legs, chest pains, palpitations, increased blood pressure and angina pectoris.

Drunk as a hot infusion, Yarrow stimulates the circulation to the skin and promotes perspiration, thus reducing fevers in colds, flu and children's infectious diseases, as well as improving immunity.

In the digestive system, Yarrow relieves poor appetite, slow digestion and promotes liver and gall bladder function through the stimulating action of the bitters. The high potassium content makes Yarrow an important diuretic that can be used to tone the urinary system in cystitis, incontinence and kidney weakness. In conditions characterized by aches and pains in the muscles and joints such as arthritis and rheumatism, an infusion drunk regularly helps to eliminate toxins and waste products.

Used externally, Yarrow is an excellent healing herb. A poultice will staunch bleeding cuts and wounds and promote tissue repair in ulcers and skin inflammations. Hildegard von Bingen recommends an eye wash for conjunctivitis; a douche or sitzbath are effective for vaginal discharges. As an ointment, Yarrow can be used to tone and strengthen weakened veins.

Emotionally, Yarrow helps to shift and balance stuck energies; used regularly, it integrates and harmonizes spiritual with emotional and physical well-being.

Dosage: Infusion: 14 g.
　　　　　Tincture: 2–5 ml.

Caution: Avoid during pregnancy. Very sensitive people can develop photosensitivity – discontinue if required.

17 | ACTION OF HERBS

Adaptogenic   helps to restore balance within the body
Alterative   helps to detoxify and renew body tissue; blood cleanser
Anthelmintic   destroys and expels worms from the digestive system
Anti-catarrhal   reduces the production of mucus and helps to remove excess from the sinuses, lungs, digestion, etc.
Anti-microbial   destroys, inhibits or resists disease-causing micro-organisms
Anti-rheumatic   relieves the symptoms of rheumatism and arthritis
Anti-spasmodic   prevents or relieves muscular spasms, cramp and mild pain
Aromatic   strong, usually pleasant smell; may stimulate the digestion, often warming
Astringent   contracts tissue and reduces secretions and discharges; drying
Bitters   stimulating tonics to digestion and liver, cooling
Carminative   eases tension and spasm in the digestive system; reduces flatulence
Demulcent   soothes and protects dry, irritated tissues, especially mucous membranes; moisturizing
Diaphoretic   promotes sweating
Diuretic   increases urination
Emmenagogue   promotes and stimulates menstrual flow
Emollient   soothes and protects dry skin; softening and moisturizing
Expectorant   expels excess mucus from the lungs
Febrifuge   reduces fevers
Galactagogue   increases the flow of breast milk
Hepatic   strengthens the liver
Hypotensive   reduces blood pressure
Nervine   exerts beneficial effects on the nervous system
Nutritive   promotes nourishment and stimulates metabolic processes
Oestrogenic   regulates secretion of oestrogen
Parturient   prepares for and eases pregnancy and child birth
Tonic   strengthens and improves the function of a specific organ, body system or the whole body; nourishes overall well-being
Vulnerary   aids healing

18 | DOSAGES

Person	Purpose	Preparation	Quantity	Frequency
Adult	*Standard*	Infusion Decoction Tincture	1 cup 50 ml or ¹/₄ cup 20 drops 5 ml*	3 x day
	Acute	Infusion Decoction Tincture	1 cup 50 ml or ¹/₄ cup 20 drops 5 ml*	Up to 6 x day
	Tonic	Infusion Decoction Tincture	1 cup 50 ml or ¹/₄ cup 20 drops 5 ml*	1–2 x day
Elderly (age 70 onwards)			¹/₄–¹/₂ of above dosages	
Baby (age 1–5)	*Standard*	Infusion Tincture	1–5 teaspoons 1 drop per year	3 x day
	Acute	Infusion Tincture	1–5 teaspoons 1 drop per year	Up to 6 x day
	Tonic	Infusion Tincture	1–5 teaspoons 1 drop per year	1–2 x a day
Children Age 5–9 Age 9–14			¹/₄ of adult dosages ¹/₂ of adult dosages	

* 5 ml = 1 teaspoon, refers to a mixture of tinctures; if taking individual tinctures, please refer to the recommended dosages in the herbal.

19 | HERBS CONTRA-INDICATED IN PREGNANCY

The following herbs should be avoided during the first three months of pregnancy, although preferably from the time of planning pregnancy to the end of breast feeding.

The list includes strong laxatives, emmenagogues and some herbs which may be prescribed by a qualified practitioner for specific complaints or during the last few weeks of pregnancy.

Common name	Latin name
Barberry	*Berberis vulgaris*
Beth Root	*Trillium erectum*
Black Cohosh	*Cimicifuga racemosa*
Blue Cohosh	*Caulophyllum thalictroides*
Cascara sagrada	*Rhamnus purshiana*
Cinnamon	*Cinnamomum zeylanicum*
Cotton Root	*Gossypium hebaceum*
Golden Seal	*Hydrastis canadensis*
Greater Celandine	*Chelidonium majus*
Juniper	*Juniperus communis*
Marjoram	*Origanum vulgare*
Meadow Saffron	*Colchicum autumnale*
Motherwort	*Leonorus cardiaca*
Mugwort	*Artemisia vulgaris*
Peruvian Bark	*Cinchona spp.*
Pennyroyal	*Mentha pulegium*
Partridge Berry	*Mitchella reperis*
Poke Root	*Phytolacca americana*
Rue	*Ruta graveolens*
Sage	*Salvia officinalis*

Senna	*Cassia angustifolia*
Southernwood	*Artemisia abrotanum*
Tansy	*Tanacetum vulgare*
Thuja	*Thuja occidentalis*
Thyme	*Thymus vulgaris*
Wormwood	*Artemisia absinthum*

Adapted from: Helen Stapelton, 'Women as midwifes and herbalists', in *Complementary Therapies for Pregnancy and Childbirth*, Tiran D. and Mack S. (eds) 1995.

20 INTUITIVE WORK WITH HERBS

Connecting intuitively with herbs is deeply satisfying. Not only does it link you with extensive herbal traditions but it is also an effective way to discover which herbs are particularly suitable for you and your needs.

Below are some questions which you may wish to ask yourself to facilitate the flow of your intuition by giving it direction. While such an exercise may seem difficult initially, it becomes easier with practice. Over time you are likely to develop your own ways of working.

The exercise

Choose an uninterrupted time and prepare a standard infusion; you may wish to light a candle; sit comfortably; sip your infusion slowly while focusing on the infusion and on yourself. After about 5–10 minutes you may want to record your experiences; these can later be compared with information found in a herbal book.

The exercise can also be done by communicating with a plant in its natural habitat. Adapt the questions as appropriate.

■ Take note of your infusion
  – What colour is it?
  – What is its aroma?
■ On slowly drinking the infusion
  – What does it taste like?
  – What is the texture?
  – What effects does it have on the tongue and in the mouth?

■ Where in the body can you feel the infusion?
  - General: Upper/lower body, centre/extremities, deep/surface, left/right
  - Head: forehead, temples, nose, ear, cheeks
  - Neck/chest: throat, shoulders, lungs, breats, heart
  - Abdomen: stomach, small/large intestine, spleen, pancreas, kidneys, liver/gall bladder
  - Pelvis: bladder, womb/ovaries, vagina/vulva, penis/testes
  - Extremities: fingers, hands, arms, toes, feet, legs
■ What effects and/or feelings do you experience while drinking the infusion?
  - Is it uplifting, grounding, relaxing, stimulating, irritating, tingly, expanding, nourishing, neutral?
  - What is its quality? Drying, cooling, warming, moisturizing, neutral.
■ How would you use this plant?
  - Would you use it for physical, emotional, mental and/or spiritual well-being?
  - Would you use it internally or externally?
  - For what kind of complaint may it be helpful?
  - What kind of person would most benefit – young or old, male or female, weak, nervous or tense?
  - Could it be contra-indicated? Pregnancy, age, poor general well-being
■ What types of preparation could be suitable?
  - Internal – infusion, food, tincture, syrup
  - External – a bath, inhalation, compress, ointment
■ Do you have any other associations?
  - Would it be suitable for you?
  - Possible combination with other plants
  - astrological sign

APPENDIX 1: SELF-CARE

Assessing well-being

To maintain well-being requires that we observe and collect personal information, learn to interpret and organize it and act accordingly.

We tend to be well when we are in tune with ourselves – our body, emotions, needs, desires, our inner and outer rhythms. By contrast, when unbalanced or ill, we tend to feel unfocused and out of touch with ourselves.

It takes some commitment to develop the routine of self-observation and awareness and to move away from the reliance on supposed experts.

One way to monitor well-being is to ask oneself regularly (and record the answers):

- How am I feeling today?
- How did I sleep?
- How is my energy?
- How is my appetite?
- Am I eating well/appropriately?
- Do I crave sugars, carbohydrates, stimulants?
- Do I drink enough fluids?
- Do my bowels move easily and regularly?
- Is my breathing regular, deep and flowing?
- How is my skin, hair, nails?
- Where am I in my menstrual cycle?
- Do my eyes feel clear?
- Do my joints move comfortably?

■ Do I hold tension in my body? If so, where?

■ Do I enjoy and look forward to my commitments?

■ How do I relate to others?

■ Do I have space and time to myself?

■ When did I last do a breast/testes examination?

The more frequently you ask yourself these kinds of questions, the more detailed and familiar will be your health portrait. This will allow you to notice changes early in any process and act accordingly.

The best medicine is preventative – ranging from adjusting your diet, taking suitable exercise and making time for rest and relaxation as soon as you notice changes in your body's messages. Simple herbal infusions can be strengthening and facilitate healing, although they are no substitute for consistent self-care.

Assessing ill-health

Whether your illness is acute or chronic, precise information is essential in order to assess the problem and plan appropriate strategies.

Ask yourself (and record the answers):

■ What exactly is the problem?

■ When did it start and how is it progressing?

■ Is there any pain? What type? Where? When?

■ Is there any discharge (e.g. from the skin, the respiratory, digestive, urinary, reproductive systems)?

■ Observe other changes: appetite, skin (colour, texture, eruptions), temperature, weight changes, energy levels.

■ What makes you feel better? Worse?

After gathering detailed information about your well-being at a particular point in time, plan your treatment carefully:

■ Consider your diet, exercise and rest.

■ Cut down on emotional and physical stresses.

■ Decide on the most suitable herbs and their form of application (internal, external) to ease symptoms and to support the body to heal itself.

■ Take only the recommended dosages.

■ Write down what you do and take, including changes in your prescriptions, and monitor effects and progress.

■ Be realistic in your expectations.

■ Allow time for convalescence before taking on full commitments again.

■ Seek professional help in:
  – high fevers, especially in babies and young children
  – sudden changes in the condition
  – cases of doubt.

Signs of a body under pressure include:

■ frequent infections

■ pain and strain in any part of the body

■ skin irritations

■ discharges from any part or opening of the body

■ fatigue, anxiety, irritability

■ mood swings, lack of concentration

■ depression

■ sleeping problems

■ food intolerance or allergies

If appropriate, plan a self-care programme to strengthen immunity and well-being (see Immune system).

APPENDIX 2: FIRST AID KIT

Herbs can be used to treat minor accidents as much as everyday ailments. Here are some suggestions for herbs to have at hand to address your and your family's daily well-being. Make any adjustments to suit your particular health patterns.

The following herbs will help you deal with many situations arising in the average household: minor infections, coughs, colds, fevers, skin rashes, swollen glands, digestive upset, acute menstrual pains, sleeping problems.

Try to respond promptly to any health changes as the aim is to help the body to heal itself and therefore to prevent ill-health rather than to cure disease (see also Appendix 1).

Dried or fresh herbs

Chamomile
Garlic
Ginger
Lavender
Marigold

Peppermint
Sage
Thyme
Vervain
Yarrow

Tincture

Echinacea: Use internally to help the body deal with any infections; externally to bathe cuts, wounds, abrasions.

Ointments

Marigold or Ribwort: For all minor cuts, grazes, wounds etc.
Comfrey: For bruising, sprains, fractures.

Oils

St John's Wort: For bruises, sprains, nerve pains, cuts, abrasions, burns including sunburn, ear infections.

Essential oil of Lavender: Use neat: for skin rashes, burns (including sunburn), wounds, insect bites, toothache. As inhalant or in the bath: for agitation, headaches, stress, sleeping problems, respiratory infections, digestive upsets.

In a compress: for sprains and bruises.

In a massage oil: for relaxation, period pains, digestive tension.

Miscellaneous

Rescue Remedy (Bach Flower essence): Use for any physical or emotional shock, trauma, accident.

Rescue Remedy diffuses extreme emotions in adults and children, helps with exam stress and in panic situations. A single drop often settles a distressed baby or toddler. Also works wonders when repotting plants.

Herbs	Acute Infection	Fever	Low Immunity	Asthma	Catarrh	Cold	Cough	Earache	Infections	Acidity Inflammations	Constipation	Diarrhoea	Flatulence	Nausea/Vomiting
	Immune System			**Respiratory system**						**Digestive system**				
Agrimony	●		●						●	●		●		
Bearberry	●													
Borage		●	●						●	●		●		
Burdock			●	●							●			
Celery													●	●
Chamomile	●	●		●	●	●	●	●	●	●	●	●	●	●
Chaste Tree														
Cinnamon	●	●	●		●	●	●		●	●		●	●	●
Cleavers	●				●			●	●					
Comfrey							●		●	●		●		
Cramp Bark				●			●							
Dandelion			●								●			
Echinacea	●		●		●	●	●	●	●	●		●		
Elderflower	●	●		●	●	●	●		●					
Fennel				●	●	●	●		●	●	●	●	●	●
Garlic	●	●	●		●	●	●	●	●		●	●		
Ginger	●	●	●		●	●	●		●		●	●	●	●
Hawthorn														
Horsechestnut											●	●		
Horsetail			●		●							●		
Hydrangea														
Ladies' Mantle	●											●		
Lavender	●			●	●	●	●	●	●	●		●	●	●
Lemon Balm		●		●	●	●	●		●	●		●	●	●
Limeflower		●		●	●	●	●		●					
Liquorice	●	●	●	●	●	●	●		●	●	●			
Marigold	●	●	●		●			●	●	●		●		●
Marshmallow							●			●		●		
Meadowsweet	●	●							●	●		●		●
Mullein				●	●	●	●	●	●			●		
Nettle			●		●		●							
Oats			●				●				●	●		
Peppermint	●	●		●	●	●	●	●	●	●	●	●	●	●
Raspberry							●		●	●		●		●
Red Clover	●			●	●		●		●					
Ribwort	●				●	●	●	●	●	●		●		
Rosemary	●	●	●		●	●	●		●			●	●	●
Sage	●	●	●	●	●	●	●		●					
Skullcap				●			●	●				●	●	●
St John's Wort	●							●	●					
Thyme	●	●	●	●	●	●	●		●			●	●	●
Vervain	●	●	●	●		●	●		●	●	●		●	●
Willow	●	●										●		
Wood Betony				●			●		●		●	●		
Yarrow	●	●		●	●	●	●		●					

Herbs	Circulatory system						Urinary system		Musculo-skeletal system	
	Anaemic	Arterio-Sclerosis	Heart\circulation	Lymphatics	Palpitations	Varicose veins	Cystitus urethritus	Water retention	Arthritis	Sprains
Agrimony							●			
Bearberry							●			
Borage					●					
Burdock	●			●		●			●	●
Celery				●			●	●	●	
Chamomile			●		●				●	
Chaste Tree								●		
Cinnamon			●				●			
Cleavers				●			●	●	●	
Comfrey	●									●
Cramp Bark		●	●		●					
Dandelion	●			●		●		●	●	
Echinacea				●			●			
Elderflower			●					●		
Fennel							●	●	●	
Garlic		●	●				●			
Ginger			●				●		●	●
Hawthorn		●	●		●	●		●		
Horsechestnut		●	●			●				
Horsetail	●						●	●	●	
Hydrangea							●	●	●	
Ladies' Mantle							●			
Lavender			●		●				●	●
Lemon Balm			●		●					
Limeflower		●	●		●			●		
Liquorice							●		●	
Marigold		●		●			●	●		
Marshmallow							●			●
Meadowsweet		●							●	
Mullein							●		●	
Nettle	●	●		●			●	●	●	
Oats	●	●	●				●		●	
Peppermint			●						●	
Raspberry							●			
Red Clover				●			●		●	
Ribwort							●			●
Rosemary	●		●		●					
Sage										
Skullcap			●		●		●		●	
St John's Wort			●		●	●			●	●
Thyme							●		●	
Vervain			●		●				●	
Willow									●	
Wood Betony			●		●	●		●	●	
Yarrow		●	●		●	●	●	●	●	

	Nervous System				Skin					Endocrine system	
Herbs	Headaches	Insomnia	Loss of vitality/ Depression	Stress/Tension Anxiety	Acne	Cold sores	Cuts/grazes/ wounds	Eczema	Heat rash	Adrenal Exhaustion	Pituitary Imbalance
Agrimony						●	●		●		
Bearberry								●			
Borage			●	●				●		●	●
Burdock					●			●			
Celery			●	●						●	
Chamomile	●	●		●		●	●	●	●		
Chaste Tree					●					●	●
Cinnamon			●								
Cleavers					●			●	●		
Comfrey			●				●	●			
Cramp Bark				●							
Dandelion		●			●			●			
Echinacea					●	●	●	●			
Elderflower											
Fennel			●								
Garlic					●	●	●				
Ginger			●	●						●	
Hawthorn		●	●	●							
Horsechestnut											
Horsetail							●				
Hydrangea								●			
Ladies' Mantle							●				
Lavender	●	●	●	●	●	●	●	●	●		
Lemon Balm	●	●	●	●	●	●		●			
Limeflower	●	●	●	●							
Liquorice			●	●				●		●	●
Marigold					●	●	●	●	●		
Marshmallow							●				
Meadowsweet							●				
Mullein							●				
Nettle			●		●		●	●			
Oats	●	●	●	●				●		●	
Peppermint	●		●						●		
Raspberry											
Red Clover					●			●			
Ribwort							●		●		
Rosemary	●		●				●			●	
Sage			●	●			●			●	●
Skullcap	●	●	●	●							
St John's Wort	●	●	●	●		●	●				
Thyme			●			●	●			●	
Vervain	●	●	●	●			●	●		●	
Willow	●						●				
Wood Betony	●	●	●	●				●			
Yarrow							●				

Herbs	Reproductive system – Male		Reproductive system – Female						
	Benign Prostate Enlargement	Prostatitis	Breast cysts	Heavy Periods	Irregular Cycle	Menopause	Painful Periods	PMS	Vaginal/Vulval Infections
Agrimony									
Bearberry		●							
Borage			●	●	●	●	●	●	
Burdock									
Celery						●			
Chamomile						●	●	●	
Chaste Tree			●	●	●	●	●	●	
Cinnamon				●		●	●	●	●
Cleavers	●	●	●						
Comfrey									
Cramp Bark				●		●	●	●	
Dandelion						●		●	
Echinacea		●							●
Elderflower									
Fennel					●	●		●	
Garlic		●							●
Ginger							●		
Hawthorn						●			
Horsechestnut	●			●		●			
Horsetail	●	●		●					
Hydrangea	●	●							
Ladies' Mantle			●	●	●	●	●	●	●
Lavender						●	●	●	●
Lemon Balm						●	●	●	●
Limeflower						●	●	●	
Liquorice						●		●	
Marigold	●	●	●	●	●	●	●	●	●
Marshmallow		●							●
Meadowsweet									
Mullein									
Nettle	●	●	●	●		●			
Oats						●		●	
Peppermint									
Raspberry			●	●	●	●	●	●	●
Red Clover		●	●	●	●	●	●	●	
Ribwort		●							●
Rosemary						●			
Sage			●	●	●	●	●	●	●
Skullcap						●	●	●	
St John's Wort		●					●		
Thyme		●							●
Vervain						●	●	●	
Vitex			●	●	●	●	●	●	
Willow					●				
Wood Betony						●		●	
Yarrow		●	●	●	●	●	●	●	

APPENDIX 4:
USEFUL RESOURCES

■ For general information on all aspects of herbal use, including medicinal, culinary and the growing of herbs, contact:

The Herb Society
Deddington Hill Farm
Warmington
Banbury OX17 1XB
Tel: 01295 692000
Email: email@herbsociety.co.uk
Website: www.herbsociety.co.uk

■ To buy medicinal herbs, check your local healthfood shop or contact the following for mail order service:

G. Baldwins and Co.
173 Walworth Road
London SE17 1RW
Tel: 0207 703 5550

■ For a list of qualified medical herbalists, contact:

The National Institute of
   Medical Herbalists
56 Longbrook Street
Exeter
Devon EX 6AH
Tel. 01392 426022

■ For information on training to become a professional herbalist, contact the Herb Society or the National Institute of Medical Herbalists (contact details given above).

Australia

Australian Herb Society Inc
P O Box 110
Mapleton
Queensland 4560
075 446 9243
075 446 9277

Canada

Canadian Association of
   Herbal Practitioners
921 17th Avenue
Calgary
AB T2T OA4

New Zealand

Herb Federation of New
   Zealand
P O Box 4055
Nelson South
03 546 9121
03 546 9121

USA

American Herbalists Guild
P O Box 70
Roosevelt
UT 84066
435 722 8434
435 722 8452
ahgoffice@earthlink.net

INDEX